Thank-you for your help with a Klara

THE PURPLE WAVE

ANCIENT SCIENCE~MODERN TECHNOLOGY, A MARRIAGE MADE IN HEAVEN

a true story by
KLARA REID

The Purple Wave
Copyright © 2020 by Klara Reid

All rights reserved. No part of this publication may be reproduced, distributed, or transmitted in any form or by any means, including photocopying, recording, or other electronic or mechanical methods, without the prior written permission of the author, except in the case of brief quotations embodied in critical reviews and certain other non-commercial uses permitted by copyright law.

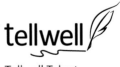

Tellwell Talent
www.tellwell.ca

ISBN
978-0-2288-1096-4 (Paperback)
978-0-2288-3194-5 (eBook)

To all Men & Women,
Mothers & Fathers

who are fighting the good fight,

by living exemplary lives

to keep their Families

Physically, Mentally &
Morally Healthy!

TABLE OF CONTENTS

ACKNOWLEDGEMENTS vii

FOREWORD..ix

PRAISES xi

DISCLAIMER xv

MEET THE AUTHOR xvii

THE TRUTH AND NOTHING BUT THE TRUTH................................xxiii

Chapter 1   THE RIGHT TO SPEAK 1

Chapter 2   DON'T BE FOOLED! 6

Chapter 3   CHANGE IN DIRECTION 14

Chapter 4   LET'S TALK.. 18

Chapter 5   THE DEAL OF THE CENTURY......................... 23

Chapter 6   WHAT DO YOU BELIEVE? 34

Chapter 7   BACK TO ORIGIN....................................... 41

Chapter 8   BORN TO LOVE 51

Chapter 9   DEAR STRESS, LET'S BREAK UP!..................... 55

Chapter 10   THE EVIDENCE IS PILING UP......................... 61

Chapter 11   THE LIGHT.. 69

Chapter 12   NUMBER ONE 76

Chapter 13   THERE IS A WAY 84

Chapter 14   FOCUSED OR NAÏVE? 94

Chapter 15   A MODERN-DAY NIGHTMARE...................... 104

Chapter 16   LESSONS FROM HISTORY 112

Chapter 17	WHAT? A HEALTH MACHINE?................................ 118
Chapter 18	THE ESSENCE 124
Chapter 19	BIOMIMICRY 135
Chapter 20	SCAM ARTISTS.. 140
Chapter 21	MODERN DAY HERO 144
Chapter 22	DEATH TO POISONS! 148
Chapter 23	PEE, STRUCTURE AND OTHER MIRACLES.............. 155
Chapter 24	PEE AND POO EVERYWHERE! 167
Chapter 25	KILLER HABITS 175
Chapter 26	CRAZY OR THIRSTY CHILDREN? 181
Chapter 27	BUSINESS AS USUAL, OR SOMETHING EXTRAORDINARY?.... 187
Chapter 28	PRICE OR VALUE? 196
Chapter 29	YOUR HEART AND THE MEDIA.............................. 202
Chapter 30	HER MEMOIR... 210
Chapter 31	GENIUSES.. 216
Chapter 32	PLACEBO?.. 222
Chapter 33	WATER BOOM 229
Chapter 34	FREED BY RESTRICTIONS?.................................... 233
Chapter 35	WHERE EVERYTHING STARTS 244

EVERYTHING YOU NEED 255

REFERENCE LIBRARY 270

ACKNOWLEDGEMENTS

Just like a marvellous concert, or a winning game at the Olympics, this book could not have been born without a fantastic group of people contributing to its creation. Without the love I received, the help I was given, the demonstrations I attended, the beautiful conversations I've had with many, the celebrations I was part of, the inspiration (thank you, Jehovah] and the love and help I got from my husband Fred, this work wouldn't have happened nor would it make sense.

Words can't express the gratitude I feel towards Sabine and Roger. I am grateful for mentors I could learn from: Gail and Paul, Rochelle and Wade. I am blessed with the best team, I love you all, you all get it! You embraced Kangen Water® and you are enjoying the benefits. This book is for your family members, your new prospects and friends who are still 'thirsty' or want to learn about the best water on Earth.

This book is for all the special people who will take the time to read it.

Thank you, Mr. OHSHIRO, Mr. ISOBI and Dr. FILTZER

I am grateful for this 'hard to find' craftsmanship, the people who produce these marvellous machines and the hard-working Staff of all Enagic® offices around the globe. We appreciate your expertise, help, hard work and kindness.

FOREWORD

Beyond a doubt, Klara Reid's book "The Purple Wave" was a sheer delight to read. Her care and compassion are evident in every chapter, while her 'in-your-face' attitude shines through when addressing the state of our 'sick care' conglomerates. Klara tells it how it is – with a steady dose and diet of how she believes it should be.

Her knowledge and understanding of ionized water are very deep, particularly Kangen Water®, yet she presents it to the reader in a simple, straightforward way that all will be able to understand. Her passion for this water and belief that everyone needs it is spot on. I have been studying the science behind ionized water and researching its effectiveness in the population for over a decade now – and I believe Klara knows more than me.

Klara holds absolutely nothing back as she 'surfs' this Purple Wave. Her personal testimony is gripping, and it adds first-hand anecdotal evidence that becomes empirical in nature when combined with the thousands upon thousands of stories that many of us have heard and been part of regarding this water that truly works on the epigenetic level in our bodies. And that's exactly why it does what it does. And Klara knows that beyond question.

Thanks, Klara. I am honored to know you and endorse your work.

Bob Wright
Director and Founder- American Anti-Cancer Institute/
International Wellness and Research Center
Author, *Killing Cancer – Not People*

PRAISES

It is a great honour that I have been asked to endorse Klara's book, "The Purple Wave." I have known Klara only for a short time, but I can attest that she is a genuine person who cares deeply for people and the world we live in today. She invites us to join her and lays bare the facts and fiction about ionised water, especially Kangen Water®, with much confidence and humour. Her book reinforces the fact that we can live a 'life without illness'.

Dr. Danya Liu, M.D.
CEO, Awesome Health Ltd.

Klara's book; "The Purple Wave" is a passionate and bold deliverance of eye-opening information on the profound effect of clean ionized water on treating chronic illnesses. This book shines a light on 'lost' information about water as medicine. A must read for those that are interested in living a longer, healthier life without needless suffering by simply turning on the tap! (Of ionized water of course!) Klara's authentic, humble and sarcastic writing style makes this book a fun read and relatable resource for those wanting a deeper understanding of how something as simple as the right kind of water can be the answer to a flourishing body and mind. A real no nonsense approach that brings water back to the surface rivaling modern medicine, as a primary treatment for optimal health.

Dr. Michelle J. Salga,
Naturopathic Doctor and
Bio-identical Hormone Therapy Practitioner

I feel blessed to know Klara as she introduced me to this fantastic hexagonal, crystal water. Thank you! I feel honoured to write what I think about this amazing book!

It was a pleasure to read the book "The Purple Wave." Klara demonstrated so much passion and enthusiasm to 'wake people up' in order to reach a higher level of health and wellness, called 'Vitality'. The chapters flow beautifully and smoothly by keeping you captivated in every sentence. She provided us with the pure truth that kept me interested to continue reading every chapter without stopping.

This book provides you with crucial information about the most important part of your body which is essential to life: Water. Also, this book opens up your mind to question everything and gives you the possibility to increase your knowledge further when she talks about other books or research done by various doctors, which I found amazing. What I loved the most was how she built in various quotes from different authors, to divert the direction of thoughts and concepts and to support her knowledge ideas and testimonials. I highly recommend reading this fantastic book to fully understand why health should be our first priority.

You will get empowered on how to take charge of your own health, by just going back to basics and not complicating your life.

A message to all, from Aurelia: All people are the chosen people, may we care for each other and allow kindness and love to unite us all, on this beautiful planet Earth! Be the change you want to see in the world!

Aurelia Vida
Registered Nurse/ Holistic Health Practitioner;
Reflexology, Light and Aromatherapy

The Purple Wave proved to be a powerful and authentic testimony that did not fail to hold back on truth and passion. Klara's desire to help others overcome health trials is obvious from the start. Her energy and conviction jumped through the pages as though it were, fittingly I might add, a splash of water waking me from my slumber.

While today's world brings many conveniences and communication platforms that allow for exchange and dialogue, it also necessitates the discernment to sift through the nonsense with which we are bombarded. Especially true this is for the realm of healing. Klara helps those who are seeking by casting aside the confusion and shining a light on the simplicity of vitality.

Klara shares from her heart how the power of this water has helped her to rediscover her innate wellness while also igniting her calling to advocate for what is true. She speaks the language of love and gratitude while not yielding to the pressures of the masses. Without hesitation Klara calls out those who intentionally mislead and offers comfort and direction for those who are seeking.

The Purple Wave is a must read for anyone looking for clarity on one of the most important foundations of health. The courageous will take responsibility for their health and transform their life by opening their heart to Klara's offer of hope. Let go of what has come to pass and cast your eyes toward that which is possible for those who earnestly seek. You will surely be rewarded by stepping through this door of opportunity!

Byron Scheffler
President, Inherent Wellness Inc.

Hi Klara, so between everything that is going on in my life at the moment I managed to finally finish reading your book. I thank you and I'm honored to have been one of your chosen you shared it with. Each page showcased who you are as a person: smart, funny, honest, passionate about what you believe in.

Your love for teaching and sharing your knowledge & wanting to reach out & help people in need with health issues shines through. Every quote was bang on as to what the subject matter was. I had a hard time putting it down & can't wait until it's published so I can buy my many copies to share with everyone I know. By far the best book I've read thus far on the importance of water & health. BRILLIANT!!!!

Love Heather xoxo

Heather Goodhope,
Global Ambassador for Enagic, BC, Canada

DISCLAIMER

The information contained herein has not been evaluated by the United States Food and Drug Administration (FDA), the Canadian Food Inspection Agency (CFIA) or Health Canada/Santé Canada.

This information is not meant to prevent, diagnose, treat or cure any disease! Individuals suffering from any illness should consult with a good physician of their choice or their health care provider.

The information in this book is fully recognised by the author who accepts full responsibility for its use and content. While we have taken every precaution to ensure that the entire content of this book is accurate and current, errors might occur. All the ideas communicated throughout the book are general in nature and should not be considered to be legal, medical, consulting, sales or any other professional advice.

In all cases you should consult with a professional advisor familiar with the particular factual situation concerning specific matters before making any decisions.

For the sake of disclosure and to be completely honest with everyone who might be reading this book: I have been an independent Enagic® distributor since 2012. Everything I have written is coming from my own independent personal study, experience and books I have read.

This work has not been examined, approved or authorised by Enagic® as a company or otherwise. I take full responsibility. All the opinions expressed in this book are solely my own.

The author is taking full responsibility and states that the company Enagic® is not responsible in any way, nor has anything to do with this book.

MEET THE AUTHOR

Who is Klara, you might ask, as I am not known as a writer, neither am I famous or infamous, at least not yet. (Who knows what's going to happen in the future?) All my life, I believed that anything is possible.

I was born on December 17th, 1954 in Szekelyudvarhely, Transylvania, Romania, where I still have two brothers and numerous relatives. We lost our parents in their sixties. My mother-tongue is Hungarian, but one of my grandfathers was originally an Austrian German (Schwarzenberger).

I left a fully blown communist Romania in 1985. We, as a family immigrated to Canada in 1987, after spending sixteen months in Israel. Two immigrations in less than two years. Not an easy task, but the experience was priceless.

Presently I live in beautiful British Columbia, Canada. The reason I moved 'to the end of the world' was initially because my health was so fragile around age forty that I could only breathe and 'survive' in the pine forests of this beautiful province, surrounded by nature. I consider BC my home, my refuge, my favourite place on Earth. I went through great health challenges for forty-five years which are now solved naturally with very little effort or cost. I feel great and I am very grateful for everything that happened in my life. The time is here for me to give back.

I am not a medical practitioner, nor do I ever want to be one. I believe that we should and must help others to get better from their ailments for 'free'. Suffering is unnecessary and unacceptable to me. I was a lifelong 'patient' until I became my own 'doctor'. I did that to survive. Because of the many years during which I avoided drinking water I became 'the poster child' for Involuntary Chronic Cellular Dehydration. **Kangen Water® changed my life.**

With my husband Fred, we are blessed with four amazing, healthy children, and two beautiful grandchildren.

Our grandchildren have smart-parents, not smart-phones who ensure they spend most of their days outside.

We opened our home six years ago to help people learn about Kangen Water® through information and otherwise. We are Certified Trainers for Enagic® and we mentor people all around the globe. In 2014 I became the first Canadian Ambassador for the American Anti-Cancer Institute as I found the AACI to be the one non-profit organization worthy of my talents and effort. I am not an expert in health; I just love people, often with 'tough love' and I tell things as they are as I am convinced that most other kinds of love are harmful.

"The Purple Wave" contains my true story. It is also filled with valuable information but ultimately it is a tribute to this therapeutic tool, called Kangen Water®. I hope that you will enjoy the book and you will get the help you need or you are looking for. I pray that you will give a serious thought to water! Your body will tell you if Kangen Water® is good for you. Horses drink six times more Kangen® than regular water. I think this very fact says it better than I can.

People don't necessarily have the intuition of animals. There are quite a few who are suspicious and skeptical when it comes to water. At the same time, they will accept synthetic drugs with no questions asked. We often say: "You can bring a horse to water but you can't make him drink". Unfortunately, this is still true today! When are we going to learn?

SO,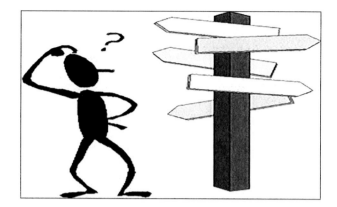

WHAT'S ALL THE HYPE ABOUT KANGEN WATER®?

Do you know what it is and where it came from?

Besides the experts who participated in creating this water, and the thousands of doctors who are on board with it, a very few might know something, others have 'heard' about it ... but the majority doesn't truly understand this 'phenomenon'. I am the proud owner of not one but two SD-501® ionizers and I have been faithfully using the different grades of water, every day, all day long, since April, 2012.

This is how I see it: to really 'get it', you need to see the 'bigger picture'! That involves the truth about tap water quality, plastic water, additives, the underlying causes of chronic illnesses, the dangerous habit of not drinking water, involuntary cellular dehydration (the real 'cancer' of society) and the insane amount of health issues we are dealing with today.

The list of 'replacements' of water is growing, causing more and more problems. This book is for those who are ill or suffering with pain, having a hard time understanding Kangen Water®, have never heard about it or aren't seeing the...

BIG PICTURE

"Seeing the bigger picture opens your eyes to what is the truth."

WADADA LEO SMITH

"TO UNDERSTAND WATER, IS TO
UNDERSTAND
THE COSMOS, THE MARVELS
OF NATURE ITSELF."

MASARU EMOTO

PREFACE

THE TRUTH AND NOTHING BUT THE TRUTH

*"But the attitude of faith is to let go,
and become open to truth,
whatever it might turn out to be."*

ALAN WATTS

Are you open? I have this burning desire to tell you all about what I found to be true about Kangen Water® and what's not. It doesn't matter how wonderful truth is, it shouldn't be pushed down anyone's throat. That wouldn't work anyhow. We are going to start with a different and hopefully much better approach.

One of the best ways to find the truth is, I think, to eliminate the lies one by one. This will take a little work but I am up for it. Are you?

Telling the truth and sticking with it is by far less demanding than lying.

I always loved to search for the truth and proclaim it no matter what. However, that's not all that I have to say. What I really hate is 'the place' where the big fat or even the 'skinny' lies take us. That place is a very uncomfortable one and it's often dangerous. I wish more people would be interested in the truth; we would definitely have a better world. Don't you think so? "How do we get to the truth", you might ask? It is a challenge, I agree, but let's give it a try anyway.

What do you think is more dangerous? To be uninformed? Or to be misinformed? I think being misinformed is worse because a misinformed person thinks he or she knows something or perhaps everything about a subject. In my humble opinion the spread of false information and half-truths today is a bigger problem than lack of information was a century ago. Rampant misinformation today causes confusion in a way society has never seen before, largely due to the exponential growth of the Internet, Social Media, and the different manipulative news outlets.

From a health standpoint misinformation is killing us by the dozens.

Certain things are not at all what they look like. For example, just because the shelves in a grocery store are filled, it doesn't mean that we have food despite what we're told or what we think. We live in a very deceiving environment and world culture. We are mislead about 200 times a day through advertisers, corporations, 'professionals', 'friends', politicians, of course, and even family members — experts say.

To know the truth about the water or the drinks we put in our bodies however—no matter how much it is ignored in mainstream information systems—is vital, for obvious reasons.

What I found is that most of the people are just as confused, uninformed and misled as I was some time ago. There is still a lack of true information out there in the world about this vital matter and this is what prompted me to write this book.

*"There is something wonderful in seeing
a wrong -headed majority
assailed by truth."*

JOHN KENNETH GALBRAITH

If you are part of this young generation who are under forty years of age of 'Internet-raised' people (part of the unsuspecting crowds of intentional or unintentional brainwashing) you might not see the craziness, the lack of common sense or wisdom that is making life chaotic. All this is causing most people to be extremely stressed out. Some grew up with it and it's all they know. For others, like myself who knew simpler times, it is chaos. **This chaos is not entirely unintentional.**

*"If you can't convince them,
confuse them."*

HARRY S. TRUMAN

How was this chaos created? I believe, like many others, that chaos on Earth came about because we got away from nature, stepped away from the 'Intelligent Designer' and His Universal Laws. Our physical and spiritual health, our actions, our goals and desires are far from God, or 'good'.

I am concerned about this environment where just about anything goes. Too many compromises have been made and there are no clear values anymore. However, it is not worth it to criticize, we just need to make it better if we can. Unfortunately, many people these days refuse to think ahead as they are blinded by the promise of big profits.

This book is not about negative people, mistakes, ignorance or the chaos we have created. It is about unique ideas and actual solutions, which already do and will have a great and positive impact in the future.

*"Great minds discuss ideas,
average minds discuss events,
small minds discuss people."*

ELEONOR ROOSEVELT

I always hated gossip, small talk, or any form of communication, which is not beneficial. I love unique, new and exciting ideas.

Awesome ideas don't have a downside to them. They are inspirations, revelations of the truth in harmony with the universe.

If you keep reading, you will find a few of my personal experiences and some of my significant or insignificant thoughts—but mostly I would like to share marvellous ideas with you brought into existence by ground-breaking science and technology from Europe and Asia. These ideas worked so well in my life that I decided to share them with you; they are worth spreading the word about because they have important implications in solving major health and environmental issues. Many people never heard about these 'revelations', so here I am, in my new reality as a story-teller and a problem-solver at the same time, writing for those who prefer natural, logical or common sense in life.

By looking at many different perspectives, we all get educated, have some fun, and hopefully don't miss the mark.

We should avoid repeating the mistakes of history! The insane 'revolution in cuisine', the convenience of processed foods (deprived from nutrients, replaced with man-made chemicals), industrialised farming with tons of antibiotics, hormones and drugs and this 'aggressive' agriculture with poisons everywhere just about destroyed our health. By the time we came to understand the consequences, the damage had been done. Most of us are aware of obesity, the 'heart issue', the 'mind issue', diabetes, cancer and more. Our overall health and longevity have been seriously compromised.

"Do you know what breakfast cereal is made of?
It's made of all those little curly wooden shavings
you find in pencil sharpeners!"

ROALD DAHL

Funny but not far from the truth. Seriously! What happened with the food supply should not happen with the water! Oh, I have bad news; It is already happening and it will be much more devastating than the previous 'adventure' mentioned above.

Now we are replacing 'what we are made of' with man-made poisons! (We are 75 percent water!)

This will become very clear to you later but think about it for a moment. Are you surprised that you are sick or not functioning well?

The time has arrived to consider the consequences of these corporations such as bottling companies, pharmaceutical companies, dog food manufacturers, those who are tampering with our food supply and the producers of toxic chemicals.

We have to do something as the time is quickly approaching when there will be no turning back!

We have to reassert our role in creating our own health.

We perhaps need to reassess our entire path for the future!

I think every 'water product' sold should come with a warning, even bottled water, as it is extremely acidic, oxidising and full of carcinogen particles from the plastic that holds it. I truly believe that all marketed drinks constitute a health hazard. However, you won't find any warning on the bottles that have flooded the marketplace. People continue to buy them, unsuspicious of how much they are contributing to a global disaster and they are destroying their health, as well.

We, who know about the hidden dangers, consider it our responsibility to create awareness about the impact of bottled water and help to correct this huge problem.

Here comes my warning: If you cannot handle honesty and truth, please do not read this book! Today's newscast might be a better choice for you. Yes. You will have to put up with my personality but hopefully my sarcastic 'style' and the frequent quotes will help me get my message across with fewer words.

In this book, I would like to achieve three things:

1. To start a conversation that matters.

2. To paint the 'Big Picture'.

3. To transmit our passion and excitement, contagious enough that it has become a global movement, a 'tsunami', if you will.

That having been said, are you ready for the best news out there?

Once I heard something like this: "The truth is simple and beautiful. It's sad that often it is kept from us." I consider this an adage for all of us to meditate on... Did you know that the truth is often kept from us? This bothers me a lot, because "the mightiest armour, the strongest shield is the revealed truth". Wouldn't it be interesting and beneficial then if we could reveal some of these hidden truths?

"Sometimes people don't want to hear the truth because they don't want their illusions destroyed."

NIETZSCHE

Ouch! Uncle Nietzsche, you are a nasty boy!

I am an optimist. I think that my readers want to hear the truth.

With all seriousness, I would like to say that it is a privilege to know about this information. Many crave change but have no idea how they can turn around and make things better for themselves and/or others.

With Kangen Water®, things are changing, a new door just opened towards a better future and you can totally be part of it. You can turn your life around. There are wonderful things happening 'behind closed doors.' There are tools you might not have, or missed. I did not know anything about any of this, either. The way I learned about it was sudden, unexpected, surprising and absolutely fascinating.

It all started in 2012 when I had a breakthrough, which not only changed my health - huge in itself - but it changed the entire course of my life. My priorities, my lifestyle, my perspective, the functioning of my brain, even my profession changed. I gained a zest for life, something I thought was a myth. My energy level went nuts. I feel thirty years younger than I did seven years ago and I love it.

This is what I call Vitality. Being alive isn't enough. I hope you agree that the quality of life is more important than the length of life. Today, I can mentally and physically challenge myself and others, younger than myself, in business, at the gym, even in the classroom.

I call this Physical and Mental Performance.

*"I intend to live life,
not just exist!"*

GEORGE TAKEI

At this point I should stop bragging and ask you: How do you perform in your everyday life? We all want to and should contribute to society. We should be givers, as well, not only takers. That would change everything. Are you able to do so? What is your point of view when it comes to your mental and physical health, the most precious things you can possess?

Oh, you don't have an opinion? Perhaps you are thinking: no one is ever going to ask me that! You might be the person who never thought about taking health matters into your own hands. Should we do that? Isn't that the job of the doctors?

Doctors most certainly have a place in our society. I love great doctors and respect the profession. But they are not 'gods'... Perhaps it might be a good idea for you to start caring for your own self. You don't have to wait until someone starts a conversation with you or you are 'diagnosed' to take control of your priorities. People seem to forget that they don't necessarily have to accept all the different pharmaceuticals or treatments that are offered to them.

There are options. Get to know your own body. Own your own health would be perhaps the most important one!

Some time ago, I was this extremely patient 'Patient' who spent precious time, again and again, at doctors' and dental offices, hospitals, chiropractors, emergency rooms, labs, naturopathic clinics and operating rooms.

Five surgeries and thirteen hospitalizations later, one day I said to myself: No more!

*"When you are sick of sickness,
you are no longer sick."*

CHINESE PROVERB

This was my turning point. I got really tired of being sick and not feeling well. Children usually ask again and again, after each answer they receive, "Yes, but why?" We should never stop being children, curious, naïve, sincere, with no limit to our imagination. At age thirty-eight, finally I asked the question "Why am I sick?"

I started 'thinking' and more importantly, I looked into some old books, interviewed some healers, talked to some 'ordinary' people, other than doctors and I prayed for wisdom, understanding and guidance. It came to me that I had to look for the cause of my medical problems to find answers. This changed everything, especially the direction my health was heading. I have never looked back...

"Buy truth and never sell it,
also, wisdom and discipline
and understanding."

PROVERBS 23:2

CHAPTER 1

THE RIGHT TO SPEAK

*"But how could you live,
and have no story to tell?"*

FYODOR DOSTOYEVSKY

Hi! I am Klara. Klara with a 'K'. There is not much to be said about who I am, I'd better tell you who I am not. I am not a medical professional, not even a dietician or a nutritionist; I am just a cook. I love real, fresh, natural foods without chemicals. We are not going to do any cooking right now because I need to talk to you 'heart to heart'. We will come back and step into the kitchen in the last chapter, I promise. For now, I am out of the kitchen, out of my profession, just out in the world travelling and talking to people. Not owning anything at all, not even a car after a bankruptcy, it's a huge relief! I got into this 'science thing' but wait! I am not a scientist, either. I have, however, spent thousands of hours looking into 'water science' and have done my own experiments on myself, our dog and family members over a period of seven years. Why? Because I love to be surrounded with happy and healthy people who are full of life and have a great sense of humour, people who are succeeding in all areas of life. I love strong people. **This is what I call normal.**

They say that to be able to talk about anything with authority, one must study the subject for a minimum of 6,000 hours. I did that because I realised that I can help myself and the people I love and make their lives better, so I went for it.

I ended up studying over 10,000 hours so in that sense I am 'qualified' to talk about drinking water and water drinking.

As a result I became a "professional" water drinker. This book is about how I have earned this 'designation' by drinking lots a water, after not drinking at all, for decades. This might sound boring to you but I assure you it wasn't boring for me. My life, full of struggles, became full of excitement. So, this book is kind of a horror story, with a marvellously happy ending. If you like those kinds of books, you might enjoy it. If not, you might learn a few lessons along the way. Anyhow I don't think your time will be wasted.

I always knew that I was a story-teller but I kept quiet until now as I had no story significant enough to tell.

OMG People! Now I have a story so huge that I am not sure if I am skilled enough to share it with the world, but I have to...

"There is no greater agony than bearing an untold story inside you."

MAYA ANGELOU

I hope you are not afraid of 'water talk'. Maybe you are?! Either way, let's discover together if this story has anything to do with you and each one of us, humans. Is water something we can ignore, forget or replace?

Is $H2O$ only a dry and boring scientific formula?

Water can't be 'dry', Klara! It is water!

Here we go! You see? My first mistake has just happened.

Anyway, this won't stop me, as I am determined to show you that water is not only relevant, but much more than that. Without it, we die. Wars are fought over it. It is bought and sold. It really is the essence of life. Yes, water is an absolute necessity and it can also be super-exciting. The amazing story of water runs like a river all through history.

What I have become conscious of is that we are not only spectators but active players in this story. We are definitely the beneficiaries (perhaps the essence) of the story. We are 'water beings.'

"We are the story and we are "WATER"..."

It took me years to get the 'Big Picture'. My goal is for you to get it in two or three days depending on how long it takes for you to finish reading 'The Purple Wave'.

Some don't understand the connection between water quality, health and longevity.

Lack of quality water or avoiding to drink water can ruin your life without realising it. I made the giant mistake of not understanding this 50 years ago... the exact thing many people are doing today.

So, in a sense, I am a forerunner, kind of a *'messenger'* of something eloquently called 'hydration' today, if you will.

There is another reason I have to talk about this: Dedicating as many hours as I have to studying this subject matter is very difficult for some. For most people it would be impossible. Our kids, family members, friends, clients and relatives do not have this amount of free time on their hands so hopefully I can help them find some answers.

You might be someone who also needs this information or perhaps you know someone who needs quality water.

I find that people need all sorts of details, the 'whole nine yards' about a topic, otherwise they think you are making things up.

What else can I tell you about me? I am a mother, a truth seeker and a passionate advocate for nature. Nature really needs advocates, having been silent for far too long.

I am also going to disclose some 'confidential information'. I struggled with annoying health issues most of my life. The 'Big News' is that it has been seven years since I have started managing my health on my own. This was possible only because of this tool, this new 'prescription' for health I have come across. It is a huge change for me to feel healthy and strong. I don't suffer pain any longer or spend money continuously, unnecessarily. I am amazed at how well I am functioning for my age - for any age, really. I don't do trips to hospitals and emergency rooms any more. Kangen Water® was the answer to my prayers. I don't want this to be a secret to anyone!

Great health should be a normal thing but actually it seems it isn't because almost everyone else my age - and even younger - is going in the opposite direction: struggling with flexibility, lack of energy, pain, knee/hip surgeries, diabetes, chronic conditions, auto-immune problems, sleeping and digestion issues, migraines or cancer.

People are looking for relief in all the wrong places! The majority doesn't know that...

...95% OF THE POPULATION ARE CHRONICALLY DEHYDRATED

and that has a lot to do with their misery.

The problem is that even when they hear it, they don't believe it.

Why would they? Conventional medicine is not acknowledging any of these facts. They talk about dry nose syndrome, dry eyes syndrome, dry throat, dry mouth, dry tongue syndrome, dry everything syndrome as some kind of 'disease', which has nothing to do with dehydration. People are having surgery for dry eyes so they can close their eye lids for God's sake. Crying with real tears would mean 'luxury' for some.

This is why we will have to dissect this whole controversial subject and introduce to you the solution, which is Electrolyzed Reduced Water (ERW).

The benefits of Kangen Water® (ERW) are not advertised in a traditional way of commerce but its popularity is growing with the speed of light because its amazing properties are shared by word of mouth. Kangen Water® is becoming a phenomenon as it has the potential to help every soul on Earth including our pets and the globe itself.

There is no controversy when it comes to Kangen Water® once you understand what it is.

Kangen Water® is a different concept or idea, fairly new to us who live in North America or anywhere else, but Japan. I really must do a decent job explaining it so you can grasp it. I don't mind putting some work into this as I always wanted to give back and make a difference in this world.

Almost everyone is interested in improving their health but people usually don't know where to start. I love to meet people and this is what I learned. People would give everything they have to get better once they are broken, however, only those with wisdom pay attention beforehand, invest time, money and whatever is needed to maintain their health.

The Purple Wave

Why are we talking about health again? Well, let me tell you. Albert Einstein was confronted once at Oxford when he repeated the same lecture for the second time. His response was that he would have to continue repeating his lecture every time he had a different answer. All I can do is to repeat Mr. Einstein. I have a different answer for you and this is why we must talk about health once again!

We humans are very different from each other but we all need two basic things: health and peace of mind.

This book might provide both, the health and the peace of mind you are looking for.

The Kangen® machine is already the most important appliance in the kitchens of those who know about it.

We have to spread the word and get the message across in order to stop the insanity of drinking bottled water and marketed drinks.

We also have to spread the word about how water should be everyone's focus before they focus on food! (Which has now became an obsession in the journey of looking for a solution!)

It is time to celebrate Kangen Water®! You might not agree. You might not be there yet but you will be before this story ends, at least that is what I am hoping for.

*"I do not agree with what you have to say, but
I'll defend to the death your right to say it."*

EVELYN BEATRICE HALL

CHAPTER 2

DON'T BE FOOLED!

*"There is a simple rule here, a rule of legislation,
a rule of business, a rule of life; beyond a
certain point, complexity is Fraud."*

P.J. O'ROURKE

One of the reasons I decided to touch this subject was because of its simplicity. I am not a fan of complicated stuff.

We are not sure about the science when it comes to water, but there is more happening out there than anyone would think. I will simplify these discoveries but I have to say what has to be told...!

*"Everything should be made as simple
as possible, but not simpler."*

EINSTEIN

We are not aware but we lose a lot of water every day, all day and all night long. The water we lose through our skin is about a half liter they say and through our mouth just by talking we lose another half liter - unless you talk as much as my husband, Fred - in that case you lose a whole liter. LOL. So, we are not even talking about elimination through our kidneys, perspiration and whatnot, we have already lost a liter of water in only twenty-four hours. With all seriousness we should pay attention to updated information on this issue and there is more.

Recent discoveries about the significance of water and its functions in our bodies is changing society's understanding of water.

There is much more to tissue hydration than simply drinking ordinary water.

The famous Romanian scientist, Dr. Henri Coanda, (1886-1972), the 'father of fluid dynamics', a pioneer in aeronautical engineering, studied water for 60 years. He stated "You are what you drink". This is true because water affects our health more than anything else. The water in our cells and tissues, however, is very different from ordinary 'bulk' water available to us in 2020. We need to feed our cells and tissues water that is bio-available or friendly to us, so our body will recognise it and work with it. That water would make a difference in our health condition.

There is some very good water that is 'bio-available' found in nature. One example is the glacier water found high up in the Himalayas, used by the Hunza people. These people and their extraordinary health were Dr. Coanda's big discovery. They routinely live for 120 plus years, with no chronic diseases, on a high fat diet. (Imagine that!) Cancer for example is unknown to them. They live a traditional, natural lifestyle and are able to look after themselves until they die. This is the way life should be, not what we have - hooked up to tubes, in a wheelchair or moved to a facility.

What Coanda - who at age 78 had an unusually quick mind and showed a vast reservoir of life or inner energy - found out was that **this totally special water he never dealt with contained 'negatively charged Hydrogen ions' and special 'colloidal mineral clusters.'** The water because of these special properties was more functional and it "behaved differently." It was 'smaller', its clusters contained only 4-6 water molecules. Dr. Coanda concluded that this water is therapeutic, it prolongs life and prevents chronic diseases. His dream was to find the 'fountain of youth'. His lifetime ambition was to recreate the Hunza water in his lab. This discovery led to many decades of research to reproduce this water.

Today some are celebrating the result of this work, this fabulous international effort with a glass of Kangen Water®. Have you heard about this? Kangen Water® has similar qualities to 'Hunza water'. It is even higher grade than glacier water, thanks to ground-breaking technology. We will discuss why this water is indeed 'medical grade'. Muslims also understand healing/holy water. They refer to the water of Zamzam as something unique. They crave this mysterious water and love to drink it. They carry it for thousands of miles and give it as a special gift to their friends and families.

So, what is so special about Zamzam water? Everything. There is nothing ordinary about it. The miracle of how it came to being in the middle of the desert, its consistency throughout thousands of years, the beneficial qualities it has, the fact that it never dries up. The fact is, this small 5ft deep well is far away from any other source or body of water. It is self-replenishing. It is distributed worldwide. Zamzam water has scientifically been proven to possess healing qualities due to its higher content of calcium and magnesium salts and special energy to start a germicidal action. It has remained free from biological contaminants. The only problem I see is that when it is bottled it will lose some of its amazing properties. You can purchase Zamzam water imported from Mecca for $20.00 or so a bottle in Canada. Wow. I have important news for Muslims. Kangen water is as close as you can get to this water. It can also be scientifically proven to have healing properties and more.

To comprehend why we would benefit from Kangen/Hunza/Zamzam water, you need to know the truth about the root causes of chronic illnesses and body degeneration. You must understand that we are all in the same boat, you are not alone and that "the quality of ordinary water is not good enough to preserve health" according to experts who are thinking day and night about the management and sustainability of our water supply.

You need to know that our health has been politicised - and that is *not* okay!

Think about this for a moment: with all the enormous advancements in the last 100 years in every other field, why is health the only area where we are going backwards? Important questions must be answered with 100 percent sincerity!

What's curious is that more than 1000 years have passed since a great mind stated what holds true still:

> *"A complete knowledge of a thing can only be obtained by elucidating its causes and antecedents, provided of course such causes exist. In Medicine it is therefore necessary that causes of both health and disease should be determined."*
>
> **AVICENNA**

What Avicenna, this great thinker, is saying sounds logical but more importantly, it works. What is really amazing about this theory besides the fact that it's true is this: When the root cause is finally found and removed, the 'job' is almost done. The recovery is almost automatic as the body can heal itself by rebuilding its natural immune system.

This is how healing happens. I am living proof.

Causes have consequences. There are 'soft' and 'hard' causes. A soft cause might be some marital trouble or an unhealthy relationship. This usually is a prolonged stressful situation; the person feels that they can't cope with the situation and there is no way out. Another trigger can be a trauma like the death of a person or a tragedy, which the person can't deal with emotionally. We are not going to deal with the soft causes in this book. Those mostly depend on the individual; they are emotional or spiritual in nature and totally personal, meaning that there are no two cases alike. We will be focusing on the so-called 'hard causes' as the root cause of health problems of today's societies, which are almost always the major contributors of premature aging and/or the chronic conditions of the body.

What do you think? If Avicenna's theory is correct and this was known all along, how come **1000 years later, most medical practitioners are treating the symptoms and never look for the causes?**

Don't be fooled!

The causes of most major degenerative conditions are known but they are ignored!

Somehow, I always had a hard time believing that this is such a complicated matter.

Look what we have created within the medical system. It has become a money-eating monster. We spend more and more and still millions are ill. We need to 'build hospitals' for children? We have to stop pretending that this is a normal thing as it is not.

We have more pharmacies today than food markets!

This might sound unbelievable to you so let me give you an example. In Chilliwack, BC, a city of approximately 80,000 people, there are over thirty pharmacies and maybe twenty grocery stores, supermarkets, fresh food markets in total. Check it out yourself!

How did we get into this situation? I will tell you in case you don't already know. Health has become a profit-driven industry where people are taken advantage of for the sake of money.

Fifty percent of the population are on multiple drugs. This has never happened before during human history.

Why are we not asking questions? Without knowing the truth, we have no chance. **I call this now, a Global Crisis.**

"I am a firm believer in the truth.
If given the truth, they can be depended upon
to meet any national crisis. The great point
is to bring them the real facts."

ABRAHAM LINCOLN

So, let's pull up some Facts. Approximatively 5,000 souls, probably even more, commit suicide every year in Canada alone, Statistics Canada states. For example, in 2015 suicide claimed the lives of 3269 men and 1136 women. A recent study by the U.S National Center for Health Statistics found that the rate of women who die by suicide increased by 50 percent between 2000 and 2016. This happened in the USA and Canada. An extremely scary reality. I am certain that at least 80 percent of these deaths are caused by prescription drugs, particularly those that mess with the brain, such as anti-depressants or anti-psychotics. These drugs cause more profound problems than the original issue.

This is what I call crazy and unethical. What are we doing?

The Purple Wave

> *"Without ethics, man has no future.*
> *This is to say, mankind without them*
> *cannot be itself. Ethics determine*
> *choices and actions and suggest*
> *difficult priorities."*

JOHN BERGER

Because I myself experienced the effects of these drugs by taking them for five months, after an acute episode [the incident was caused by stress, lack of sleep due to marital problems and dehydration] I know it from personal experience that they cause suicidal thoughts or an urge to commit suicide, which is very difficult to resist. I cannot close my eyes and pretend that this is not happening. Only by the grace of God I am still alive, after these five months as somehow I had the wisdom to call my doctor during my planning to jump off the 14-th floor who acted immediately and took me off the drug.

An experiment was done using a tiny microchip, which was attached by researchers to different drugs to see what those drugs would do in the human system. It showed that the drug travelled all through the brain and the body and was rejected by every single cell and organ until it ended up in the liver. I found this interesting but not surprising. This story was told during an interview by the famous Sadhguru so I apologize but I could not verify its truthfulness. Sadhguru Jaggi Vasudev simply referred to as Sadhguru is a well-known Indian yogi, educator and author. He is involved in social outreach, education and environmental initiatives. He was born in 1957 and studied at the University of Mysore, India. He often talks about water and how water should be treated with respect and understanding. When I saw this interview, I looked for this story everywhere but I could not find anything about it. An experiment like this would not be public knowledge, I am sure of that. It is unfortunate that some very important information as this is kept from the public, still.

> *"When there is information there is enlightenment. When there is debate, there are solutions."*
>
> **ATIFETE JAHJAGA**

Anyhow, when a person is taking synthetic pills, how long until the liver and the kidneys say: Enough!

Yes, we have pollution and stress around us and there is also a new killer out there called EMF (Electro-Magnetic-Fog) but I continue to ask ... why are we continuously spending money on and poisoning ourselves with thousands of products created by different industries that we don't need for our existence or happiness? Integrity is gone. We are offered 'everything under the sun'. We should refuse to buy these things! Why go along with the lies and immorality of those who create these products?

We forget at times that we can leave the 'herd' as soon as we realize that it's going in the wrong direction.

Are we losing consciousness about human dignity?

Many, many questions come to my mind.

> *"Rather fail with honour than succeed by fraud."*
>
> **SOPHOCLES**

I love this country but I oppose the direction our medical system is going south as our healthcare will not pay for anything which is preventative. There are no signs for real change, no initiatives and no long-term plans to create a healthier society. Those who are not aware of how to take care of themselves are practically funnelled toward death, for free, by our unilateral medical system, which ultimately will poison them or make them dependent on these poisons. The cost of natural treatments must come from our pockets if we want to avoid health disasters. I have been there, done that. It wasn't easy.

Real, nourishing food is becoming rare and very expensive.

Today 6,000 kinds of drugs are prescribed and to 'justify' that 12,000 labels called 'diseases' have been created. We can't possibly keep up with this so I should let you know that help is here and it is exactly what we need!

> *"Our prime purpose in this life is to help others, and if you can't help them, at least don't hurt them."*
>
> **DALAI LAMA**

Almost everything from personal care and cleaning products to agents used in agriculture and the food industry is toxic. These toxins end up in our water supply. This vicious cycle was created by us, the irresponsible man. The funny thing is that it doesn't have to be this way. It makes me sick when I see what some have in the bathroom and under the kitchen sink. Bottles and bottles of chemicals. So much money wasted, so much harm caused.

The purpose of this work is to spread the word about a complete paradigm shift, which not only will help you to be healthy, but also can interrupt this vicious cycle.

We can now replace most of the chemicals we use in the household. We can be almost totally eco-friendly. It sounds 'too good to be true' or perhaps futuristic?

I think, we give up far too easy.

I would not be alive today if I would have kept doing what most of the people are doing.

Never lose Hope! "Never give up my friend until the very end!"

Kangen Water® is here!

> *"If there is magic on this planet, it is contained in water."*
>
> **LOREN EISELEY**

CHAPTER 3

CHANGE IN DIRECTION

*"The noblest pleasure is the
joy of understanding."*

LEONARDO DA VINCI

The so-called Kangen® machine, which many are inquiring about is an idea that was perfected into a medical device to help us manage our health and keep our environment safer. The problem is that it won't serve the masses unless they learn about it and use it. It is time for you to find out about the advantages of using this tool, experience the benefits of the waters and learn why you should consider owning at least one as soon as possible.

Please don't ask me the question *"If this is such a fantastic thing, why are we not told about it and why is the government not recommending it?"* Seriously?

Over forty-five years have passed since this invention. We already know that it has only positive effects on people's health and the environment. We don't need more studies and more time.

The time is now!

The Purple Wave

The 'product' of the Kangen® machine is 'Electrolyzed Reduced Water'.

During the book, I will refer to this water as "ERW"! This is not a new 'type' of water, nor is it 'alkaline water'. Knowing the truth about sodas, we don't want anything new. Enough said!

Kangen Water® has changed well over a million lives and - Get this! - there have been no side effects, no lawsuits, no insurance claims or payouts. The Kangen® machine is simple to use and it is producing five different grades of water for totally different uses. I know, I know, I thought the same thing you are thinking: Water is just water, but I also know that by setting things straight, you will realise yourself the mind-blowing mystery, art and science of water.

Why does it take so much time for something this great to be adopted by the majority? Legitimate question.

When it comes to truly amazing things, people in general are skeptical. Most 'minds' are conditioned to believe propaganda, illusions and not necessarily the truth. This contributes to the unnecessary suffering of millions. Besides, the majority is always wrong! This might sound weird to you, but try to be different, change your direction and you will be fine.

"Direction is so much more important than speed. Many are going nowhere, fast!"

UNKNOWN

High-end and revolutionary products like the Kangen® machine require education, not because of the complexity of the device, but because of the complete change in lifestyle and the endless opportunities, which can be achieved with it.

The concept of ERW is for the open-minded, especially for those who just know in their hearts that there has to be a better way.

Several times this happened during my life and it always turned out to be right. Yes, I know, I sound a lot like Simon Cowell (the biggest name in talent discovery) but it is a lot of fun to be right. Try it sometime!

You can't afford to be shy about your health. There is so much out there to see. The key here is 'Intellectual Distribution.' In case you are not familiar with the term, here it is. I have never seen an actual definition but this is what I think about it: Intellectual distribution means sharing 'Intellectual Property,' revolutionary innovations the right way. It is done by educated, brilliant entrepreneurs, who are doing a great service to the consumer. Unlike physical distribution, intellectual distribution requires courage, time investment, understanding, knowledge, wisdom, experience, communication skills, vision, even diplomacy. Thanks to these professionals, the consumer can learn about the need, the truth, the product, the advantages or disadvantages, the circumstances, the possible scams, all they need to know about a subject. Unlike during ordinary advertising, lifelong relationships are created here, reputation is at stake and real responsibility is understood and undertaken. This is important because the majority doesn't have time to read anymore. It is unfortunate because when we are hungry for knowledge, our lives improve.

The secrets of life are hidden in books. Knowledge is hidden, it always has been and that has not changed since ancient times (the best example is the Bible, of course). One might get a lot of information from the Internet but what they find is not necessarily true knowledge.

"You don't have to burn books to
destroy a culture.
Just get people to stop reading them."

RAY BRADBURY

Every person deserves the truth!

If only mothers could really hear me. If medical practitioners would only listen, they would easily understand the science leading to this discovery.

The Purple Wave

When I first heard about Kangen Water®, I became passionately curious because of my poor health. I kept hearing it in my head over and over again that: ***This new idea and technology is considered the biggest breakthrough in medicine since Fleming's discovery of penicillin and that's a long time.***

The biggest one and I did not hear about it? That just can't be! Yet, it is indeed true. OMG. Because of this amazing water, I got another chance.

We, self-centred humans, got another chance! We should influence the world, I was thinking. The thoughts going through my mind were appealing, shocking and provoking at the same time. I had many sleepless nights as I slowly came to the realisation that we can change direction regarding quite a few things which seem very important as these changes will affect our whole lifestyle. I have never been this excited about any of my purchases ever before.

We are influenced every day and the things we are being pushed to are not taking us in a direction that serves us best. Do you ever wonder about alternatives, a different path, a possible solution? Have you ever wanted to 'rebel' against things that made no sense to you? In the event that you like what you are reading, we can turn this crazy world around by starting to do things the right way! Come on aboard so we can create some ripples together....

"I alone cannot change the world, but
I can cast a stone across the waters to
create many ripples."

MOTHER TERESA

CHAPTER 4

LET'S TALK

"The best way to solve problems and to fight against war is through dialogue."

MALALA YOUSAFZAI

You might be thinking: *What war is she talking about?* **The war on your immune system!** Yes, *that* war I have the audacity to talk about. This war has been going on for a while and so many are still not realising it, which makes it even more dangerous.

Chronic illness will paralyse our society. You don't have to be an expert to see it. The root causes why so many are ill are well known. They are Dehydration, Acidosis and Oxidation, in that order. It is kind of a chain reaction, which is happening from pollution (air, water and food), stress, and a wrong lifestyle, mostly rooted in bad habits. This is it! Really? I know you are hesitant to believe me.

When I first heard this, I thought, it can't be this simple as this can be easily understood by anyone. Professionals who've spent a decade and tons of money studying can't figure out why we are sick never mind how to fix the problem so this is a bit confusing. I agree. There is something else. A special situation emerged for the first time in history and you don't

18

The Purple Wave

hear about it: **The 'Treatment' is gradually becoming the leading cause of thousands of new health problems.** Are you aware? Nowadays it is safest if you don't get 'treated'!

Over thirty years ago my Mom died as a result of taking thirteen different kinds of pills, prescribed by her physician, which she took every day. The first one was prescribed for irregular heartbeat, caused by magnesium deficiency due to stress. (We had no idea then, but I understand this today, thirty years later...) She had no other problem at the time of her first doctor's visit. She was a strong woman who never used illegal drugs, pills or alcohol. She had the same natural diet we all did and had a healthy lifestyle. Never smoked. Soon after the first two pills were prescribed, more and more problems started.

We did not make the connection between the new health problems and the growing number of medications she was taking.

We did not know what we know now. People are scared and confused about being unable to perform a normal life and this fear, this 'not knowing' just adds to the problems. We live overcomplicated lives in this 'era of controversy'. What do you expect? Simplicity? We even argue about gender, something we are born with; why would we agree on the illnesses or treatments? How about you? Are you scared? Are you depressed or concerned about your family members? Are you confused, still in the dark? Do you understand these connections?

> *"Nothing in life is to be feared,*
> *it is only to be understood. Now is*
> *the time to understand more, so that*
> *we may fear less."*
>
> **MARIE CURIE**

I can only be grateful that today I understand the cause and effect theory regarding health and the damaging things we do to ourselves. Many times, what we neglect can hurt us even more. That is logical but not always self- explanatory. Usually when something has logic to it, I get it. However, the majority are outside of this 'zone'.

What a horrendous crime was committed against the native population when slowly their traditional way of making medicine with plants and roots was lost to the medical system as we know it today. These gentle and still very effective natural remedies studied for centuries and used by the medicine man of the tribe have been replaced with synthetic, addictive pills. Should we be satisfied with this situation? I don't think so.

What I am proposing is a change in lifestyle, a switch to something that is simple and natural. Change is needed like fresh air, which we don't have any more so it is needed even more.

Those of us who understand Kangen Water® have invested our own money and time; in many cases we made huge sacrifices to get this knowledge out. We 'live' this lifestyle; we are drinking this water all day long, every day, not only recommending it to others. That is extremely refreshing, don't you think so? Did you know that 'cancer specialists' would not subject themselves to the very treatments they recommend to their patients? This is revolting to me.

I call this the ultimate hypocrisy.

According to one study published in the "Journal of Clinical Oncology," in 1987, "81% of cancer specialists would not consent to a drug trial due to the ineffectiveness of chemotherapy and its unacceptable degree of toxicity." This is what Dr. Zoltan Rona, of Toronto, Ontario, one of the most recognized physicians in Canada, stated in an interview.

I hope that by now it is obvious to you, as well, that we can't fix any of the problems with the same mindset we created them. To fix health care issues in today's society, we need to go back in time when life was less complicated.

We live in this new era of instant communication worldwide. This is great, I think. Let's use the Internet and everything we can to make great ideas known and use everything we can to make life better for all of us.

What happened in 2009 was great! Tens of millions of people in the USA and Canada avoided a disaster just by communicating openly. People got informed and refused the swine flu shot. (Smart people!)

I love open, real, honest conversations, TEDx talks, everything which is spontaneous (non-political) and uncontrolled. I love surprises, good ones of course. On talent shows the whole world can now witness when a new star comes on stage. For a while now, they are not coming out of immoral Hollywood, but from places like this tiny village in Scotland. Remember Susan Boyle? The world is changing. Believe it or not, the same is happening in the arena of healthcare. I think this is great. We can't expect real change from those within the health care system, either. An 'outsider' might become the next star of true health.

I hope that this information will cause people who bow down in front of everything 'scientific' to think twice. Not all science is pure and not all science serves the individual. Remember microwaves? Nasty science! They transform food into garbage. Hopefully they will be only a thing of the past. The mammogram, which was made mandatory thirty years ago, has been taken out for good in some countries as the results are often inaccurate and they are causing more problems than they are solving. There is so much that is questionable in the medical system when it comes to the science of it. Whistleblowers are coming out almost daily about how there is practically no true science behind most of prescription drugs.

"Nothing is more irredeemably irrelevant than bad science."

JOHN CHARLES POLANYI

I dream about a better future. Better yet, I see a greater future for most of us.

I hope this information will be a wake-up call for people who are suffering, constantly going to diagnostic testing, wasting precious time, spending money on the wrong treatments and supplements. Are you getting results? If not, why continue to do the same thing for years and just waste your hard-earned money? Our body cannot use synthetic pills! They are not 'bio-available.' Can your car run on lemon juice or vinegar? Of course not. Different design!

A great thing about the Internet is that we can learn about the different options and opinions on things, including medical issues. We can listen to experts who are fed up and finally are telling the truth, so please learn the truth about statin drugs, cholesterol medications, acid blockers, beta blockers, water pills, etc. It is all there! At least for now. We must educate ourselves and communicate so that we can see through the special interests of lobbyists, the evil out there and the manipulation of the media.

"Communication, the human connection-, is the key to success."

PAUL J. MAYER

Let's use this privilege as long as we have it. I think it's a mistake when some people isolate themselves from open communication. They become victims. You can see this by trying to get someone to an educational seminar! Eighty percent of the time they will have an excuse, something like the kid's soccer practice or ballet class, a birthday party, for example, which is the same every year anyways and besides being an ego booster, I could never understand the point. Parents are often more interested in the athletic performance than the diet or the health of the child. This is commonplace now.

Should we call this weird parenting?

CHAPTER 5

THE DEAL OF THE CENTURY

*"In a gentle way, you can
shake the world."*

MAHATMA GANDHI

We can do much, much better. I know it! Let's start with what we know for sure! Virtually all scientists and researchers in the world today agree on the theory of free radical damage and over acidity, as the main cause of degenerative illnesses. To simplify this, you just have to imagine this: our billions of cellular molecules are held together by electronic bonds. These bonds can weaken due to environmental factors (smoking, pollution, lack of sleep...etc.). What really happens is that these molecules lose an electron. This is a naturally occurring process but it can get out of control and when that happens, a chain reaction begins. These molecules want to be whole again (naturally) so they start stealing electrons from nearby healthy cells causing them to lose one of their two electrons. They will become 'free radicals.' These will cause oxidation in the body, something similar to a rusting or corroded metal or a slice of apple, which turns brown soon after we cut the fruit. To stop this, we need antioxidants or agents, which are capable to stop this oxidation. Most of the people have heard about antioxidants. Now you know why we need them.

We all agree that excess stress is bad for us and we have more and more of it. What I did not know until I started doing some 'digging' was that **dehydration is the main (underlying) stress of all stresses!**

Strange concept? We will elaborate on this theory soon enough.

Everyone is looking for a magic substance like a pill or super-food, something, which will stop these free radicals before they do damage. We are often looking for something to alkalise our over-acidic bodies. I used many different alkalising 'tools' to help me survive twenty-five years ago when I was ill. I was juicing, detoxing, taking tons of antioxidants. I did colonics, massages, 'energy treatments', which I paid lots of money for just to stay alive. These are all good but this is the hard and expensive way to get one's health back. Specific diets can be expensive and complicated. There is a better way! If we include water to the equation everything changes.

The 'magic substance' many are looking for is here and it has been from the beginning. It only needed a bit of 'fixing' as we have ruined it.

So, this new art is rooted in something very old. I know I am not clear enough, but I promise I will get it out of me soon.

My job is to reveal it to you the same way it was revealed to me by many different beautiful people and by the technology itself. It's a 'pay it forward' kind of a thing. I must find the right angle to introduce this simple 'miracle' to you so you will understand it. It's good to know the reason behind the miracle. The benefits are huge. It is truly "the deal of the century"; you just need some basic understanding to 'get it', to see that this is exactly what you need. It is definitely worth your time.

Many scientific studies have been done regarding Electrolysed Reduced/Restructured Water, or ERW for short. I am only guessing but I think that numerous archives in Japan and other countries are loaded with data. Books, scientific abstracts, articles, peer reviewed studies have been written; documentaries, sophisticated presentations have been shared on the subject. Thousands of 'demos' have been shown to the public in many different languages. This is going around the globe as we speak. There are hundreds of testimonials on YouTube, by ordinary people, whose lives have changed because of it. My goal is to offer the story to you in a way that you can grasp the essence and apply it in your own life, with the least time spent on research or doubt. I will cater to your logic ...I know you have it! I will have to leave you with no doubts at the end as this is too important.

You will hear many short stories behind the 'big story'. We will put all the pieces of the puzzle together but first I have to restore your confidence in human decency, in the goodness of the human heart and in the capability of the human mind. Yes, we live in a very deceiving world but I assure you that noble and wonderful ideas do exist, even today!

When it comes to our health, there is no such thing as the 'individual'. There is only oneness with all of us and with the universe itself. We all need each other. We all affect the other. None of us would exist or be happy without the rest. We only must recognize this. We all should work together.

Let's take better care of each other! This starts with taking care of ourselves first!

"The planet... desperately needs more peacemakers, healers, restorers, storytellers and lovers of every kind. It needs people who live well in their places. It needs people of moral courage, willing to join the fight to make the world habitable and humane."

DAVID W. ORR

Yes, we need all these things beautifully summarised and expressed by David Orr. "Moral courage" is huge in my book. In my humble opinion, lack of moral courage is what got us into trouble in the first place.

We can start our 'fight' with some bold statements. Our bodies are extremely sophisticated, you see. Science is discovering that a single cell is more complex than a man-made computer, yet the human body is relatively simple to take care of. This is good news! I trust the Creator. I can see that everything inside the body is pre-programmed! Everything happens on a cellular level. We need to learn how to be good to ourselves, how to keep our cells alive! We have a few trillion of these, I learned, so it is important to understand this concept. In the meantime, during history, this is what happened:

"Modern society has been built at random, according to the chance of scientific discoveries, and to the fancy ideologies, without regard for the laws of our body and soul. We have been the victims of a disastrous illusion—the illusion of our ability to emancipate ourselves from natural laws. We have forgotten that nature never forgives."

ALEXIS CARREL

Dr. Carrel (1873-1944), this French man-of-science, surgeon, biologist, author and professor educated at the University of Lyon was a real genius, a thinker well ahead of his time. I find his discovery fascinating. He received a Nobel Prize for keeping a culture of embryonic chicken heart, a living cell, alive in the lab for thirty-four years.

This is what he said about his findings:

"The cell is immortal. It is merely the fluid or water in which it floats that degenerates. Renew this fluid by giving the cells what they require and as far as we know, the pulsation of life may go on forever."

"Give the cells what they require" ... we must investigate this! Wow.

This is truly a 'wow' statement. Do you find this intriguing? This makes so much sense to me.

Not long ago, I read about how scientists find so-called 'Blue Zones'. Those are areas of the world where people are the healthiest and live the longest.

These areas always coincide with the places where the best quality of water is available. Always!

This can't be a coincidence and it isn't. Our cells are mostly water so it makes sense.

The body breaks down when the cells can't function properly or communicate between themselves.

Why can't they function? Two reasons only: Deficiency and/or Toxicity.

First let's look at the deficiency issue. What is 'deficiency'? What the cells need, they are not getting. Simple enough. The cells need the raw materials, which are water and nutrients plus the energy to have the job done. Water being the main thing (somewhere between 70 and

85 percent depending which part of the body we are talking about), the deficiency of water is the logical choice as the most important raw material. Most people know about nutrient deficiency so today we won't jump to number two as fast as we usually would. Not before we understand 'number one'. We got it this time. 'Dehydration' or water deficiency means not enough water or perhaps not 'the right water' in the cell. Wow, how many times I came across the deficiency issue before and I never gave a thought to water. I was in the dark. They say that it is easy to overlook the most obvious. The light regarding water deficiency will be turned on all throughout the book so we can now talk about the second raw material, which is the nutrients, themselves.

Some of the serious nutrient deficiencies are related to acidosis because the more acid we have to deal with, the more our mineral reserves will be used up in order to neutralise the acid. This will bring us back to water. Why? Because the neglect or lack of detoxing will result in accumulation of acid. To get rid of acidosis or the toxins, we need water. Finally, deficiency happens when the nutrients can't get to the cell and utilized. This theory again is taking us back to water. Why? Because water is the only means of transportation of nutrients. Are you getting it? Just as 'every road leads to Rome', everything leads to water!

> ## "Have you heard that joke about dehydration? False. Hydration is not a joke!"
>
> **UNKNOWN**

I will never forget the impressive story of Dr. Myron Wenz, a visionary and a scientist from Utah, United States. I came across this information about fifteen years ago. It was fascinating to learn by seeing this movie about him, how he tried to find nutrients to keep the cells alive in his lab by feeding them with the right 'food'. He is the founder of Gull Laboratories, which he sold for multiple millions of dollars, decades ago. He decided that instead of diagnostic testing he would spend his life and money on preventing illnesses. I see his work as continuation of the work of Dr. Carrel.

Dr. Wentz's story started when he got ill at a young age. He had heart disease in his forties. He knew that synthetic pills would not solve his problems. He witnessed his father dying of heart disease at a young age and he understood the causes of his death. He refused to take the same path. He tried everything available on the market at the time to improve his health but none of the food supplements he found were of good enough quality.

They had no *real* ingredients and of course, they couldn't keep the cells alive in his lab. Are you listening?

Dr. Wentz, who was born in 1940 and has a Ph.D. in Microbiology and Immunology, became extremely frustrated which inspired him to create the famous USANA vitamins with the right synergy and outstanding quality. USANA became world famous. He risked millions of dollars but it was the best investment anyone could make. He is considered today a titan of the industry. His vitamins helped him and me, as well. I paid a substantial sum of money for a period of twelve years and I'm glad I did so. Today, I've cut the cost to a third because I have what Dr. Wentz did not have. I have water, which will take these nutrients - not only twenty percent of them, but 100 percent of them - to the cells where they are utilized. (In the case of all supplements or drugs, the amounts are calculated for regular water absorption, which is apparently only about eighteen to twenty percent).

I love to follow people and listen to their stories. It is very different than 'advertising'. Stories are true most of the time. Commercials are fake most of the time. Big difference.

> *"If you want a happy ending, that depends of course, on where you stop your story."*
>
> **ORSON WELLES**

I know this for sure. Great, viable solutions, 'big ideas' are born only when we serve selflessly and we genuinely want to help. Then, and only then, we are in harmony with the Universe and our purpose because we are creating with love and from the depth of our hearts.

I call those ideas, the 'real deal.'

The Purple Wave

From Dr. Wentz's story, we can see how important the main nutrients truly are.

We are lacking nutrients because:

1. Our food is not adequate any more in that regard: first, we have aggressive agriculture that uses too many chemicals; second, we have brainless processing and cooking of foods.
2. Because we don't have the internal, biochemical means of transportation to get these nutrients to our cells where everything takes place.
   Why is that? Again, two reasons only:
   1. We don't drink enough water.
   2. The water we are drinking it's not functional, it doesn't have the power to do its job; it is deteriorated to that point. Mostly it just goes through us and it doesn't penetrate or absorbs into the cells (we will explore this theory further).

"Nutrient utilization is more important than just nutrient consumption." says Shan Stratton, one of my favorite nutritionists who is also advising top athletes in the United States. I agree with him 100 percent, as this explains why some are healthier even with less healthy diet than others who eat healthier but can't utilize the nutrients because of the lack of enzymes for example.

Now, let's talk about toxicity. Our bodies are overloaded with toxins from a polluted environment, compromised food supply, indigested stuff, wrong lifestyle, excess stress, which are all acid-forming, including synthetic pills, pesticides and more. One of the main reasons why the toxins will accumulate is that we don't drink nearly enough water. Water should be at least neutral or slightly alkaline but everything we drink is acidic causing acidosis in the body. The pH (acid-alkaline balance), which is very sensitive and regulates the immune system, is compromised. (We will discuss what this really means in a few minutes.) Acid is not good; in fact, it is very bad for us. Acid means oxygen deficiency in the cells.

As early as 1931, Dr. Otto Warburg (1883-1970), a German physiologist and medical doctor, stated: "All normal cells have an absolute requirement for oxygen, but cancer cells can live without oxygen - a rule without exception. Deprive a cell 35% of it's oxygen for 48 hours and it may become cancerous." Dr. Warburg's field was cell biology and he is the winner of two Nobel Prizes. I never heard his name or his significant discovery before I started to study water, alkalinity and the causes of cancer. I had to get further in my 'research' about why and how we get acidic and what else will contribute to acidosis?

It looks like our body fluids and tissues get too acidic except the blood. The blood is very unique so we have to talk about it in more detail in a little while. Did you know that all the fluids we know about are either acidic or alkaline? Only water has this unique 'personality' where it can be either acidic or alkaline. For a few decades now, we have been drinking all sorts of 'acidic garbage' and we are not conscious or aware about it. I drank mineral water for many years and had no idea how acidic it was. Bottled mineral water due to the infused carbon dioxide is as acidic as all regular sodas.

When we get sick, when we are in a 'pre-cancerous state', when we get run down, after an accident or a trauma, in a state of prolonged stress, we don't have excess energy to recover or heal. We hardly have energy to function. Often, we choose pills, the 'quick fix', to make us feel better. That pill, however, is a 'lie' aiming to fool the body but...

...The body cannot be fooled; the laws of its functioning were established a long time ago.

"The laws of nature are the laws of God,
whose authority can be superseded
by no power on earth."

GEORGE MASON

Sick or injured people would like a new body given to them as fast as passing through a drive-through but sometimes what they need is a break. We never rest anymore; we are overworked! Even cancer patients continue to hold regular jobs. They are doomed to die. I remember a time when people with cancer took two-three years off any kind of work to heal. Soon we are going to have so many ill people that we won't have enough caretakers! What then? Can you afford three years off all your activities to recover? I can't. That's why I do 'full time' on prevention!

I have tried to fool my body many times but it never worked. I always gain weight when I overeat. I can't skip sleep, either. Those who skip sleep with the help of coffee will pay the price. The body never changed, our lifestyles and environment did and that is exactly what we have to 'investigate' further. Imagine life only 100 years ago, with no coffee shops, small pharmacies using mostly herbs and natural remedies, fresh air, clean water, sunshine, no air-conditioning or fluorescent lights, natural food, no chemicals, pesticides, cell phones or chlorine. What a beautiful life that would be! The problem is that it doesn't exist any longer for the majority of people.

I would like to mention here the legitimate use of drugs and chlorine to kill pathogens. Water-borne illnesses have killed more people than anything else during history. It was necessary at one point to use chlorine in water but that doesn't mean that it is good for us. About fifteen percent of all drugs, so they say, are necessary. They have been a blessing to millions in the past and lives are saved all the time because of them. The problem is the unethical use of them, or the other 85 percent. Do you really think that getting better from being run down is as simple as taking a pill or something? Degeneration can only be stopped by faster regeneration. Pills are not a tool to achieve this task.

The body will never get better from chronic conditions without going through the pain and making the effort to restore health. One must sometimes suffer for months, if not for years, to rebuild immunity. It took me about two years to detox and regain my strength when I was terribly ill twenty plus years ago.

> *"Man cannot remake himself without suffering, for he is both the marble and the sculptor."*
>
> **ALEXIS CARREL**

Why do so many believe that their ruined health can be fixed by a pill or some other unrealistic miracle?

So, is there a future for us? I am interested in this not necessarily for myself, but for the sake of our children. I started to get involved after I came across a certain book, which caused serious sparks in my heart and made sense in my mind. It was quite shocking to recognise the 'crazy' episodes of my life labelled as mental or physical illnesses before and learn that in reality, they were mostly 'stages' of dehydration, nothing else. The author of this extraordinary book is the one-and-only Dr. Batmanghelidj.

The 'water theory' detailed in his two books, "You are not sick, you are thirsty!" and "Your body's many cries for water" is the most advanced and logical medical revelation I have ever read. It looks like I am not alone. This is what university professor, Lekan Oyedeji, from Lagos, Nigeria, has to say about this book: "I must confess, that apart from the Holy Bible, I have yet to find a book as enlightening as the above, in the breakdown of normally complex technical, scientific jargons and in the presentation of such to the previously uninformed."

> **"The reading of good books is like conversation with the finest people of the past centuries."**
>
> **DESCARTES**

How do you like these conversations? I adore these conversations from another era and enjoy them as it gives me a totally different prospective. Reading either of these two books is where you start if you want to learn about the human body and the root causes of your problems including depression. You don't have to go to university or read hundreds of books and scientific papers.

Here is another viewpoint from Dr. Geroge J. Georgiou, Ph.D. about this ground-breaking work: "Rare indeed are those books, destined to become all-time classics. Even rarer are books destined to accomplish a Paradigm Shift in any major areas of modern knowledge. Of still greater rarity are books to benefit significantly the health of countless millions of human beings, at no cost to them." "At no cost to them". Wow. This is the point I am trying so hard to make. The cost is near nothing when you improve your health by using water. The money I saved after discovering this 'secret' tool (not really a secret, it's just not discovered by the majority) adds up to huge numbers. Here, I just have told you the first secret. Get the book so you can manage your health efficiently and at no cost.

Health care doesn't have to be expensive.

We will find out soon who this amazing doctor, Dr. Batmanghelidj or Dr. 'Batman' is -as we call him- for he is an important persona in this story.

"It is very expensive to give bad medical care to poor people in a rich country."

PAUL FARMER

CHAPTER 6

WHAT DO YOU BELIEVE?

*"Sometimes your belief system is
really your fears attached to rules."*

SHANNON L. ALDER

Are we going along with a system that has not been working for us for decades because we fear change? Are we too attached to ridiculous rules? During history but especially the last 100 years, the so-called 'universal laws' got replaced with man-made rules, stupid habits and different routines, which make no sense whatsoever. None of these are a smart thing to do, in my opinion. Discipline, responsibility towards ourselves, good habits and smart therapeutic routines have been out for a long time now. Some natural therapies just started coming back.

I realised some time ago that 'the majority' are not using the 'universal solvent' in any way. Not only do we not drink enough water, but things like 'colonics' for example, one of the most cost-effective natural flushing methods, are 'out of style'. In the '50s it was common practice in western hospitals, as well to do a complete 'clean-up' when someone got 'plugged'. This doesn't happen only to the pipes in your house, you know!? This method of getting better fast and naturally was stopped and soon medications took over the most civilized part of the world. How insane! We forgot all about water. We don't even respect water.

We are too lazy to drink water. We don't want to pee *(You kidding me? That is time consuming!)* so we avoid water! *Why waste time by going to the toilet? Who can afford that?* We are rushing all the time and we are lazy.

Our laziness is driving the economy more than anything else.

We are tired to the point that we are standing in line for 'booster shots' at Starbucks or at coffee shops, daily.

We have a physically and mentally ill society.

There is a better way! This would be the natural, a quite obviously superior, way of doing things. Don't you think that natural is much easier to comprehend? Of course, it is. This is what universal means! The same obvious, boring rule for everyone - not opinions - only weird, politically incorrect, long forgotten, raw, hate provoking, 'unjust' truth!

> *"If we surrendered to Earth's intelligence,*
> *we could rise up rooted like trees."*
>
> ### R. MARIA RILKE

Let's rise up with this idea! Our theory for now is that the quality of our everyday drinking water and/or the lack of water is what is behind the tremendous increase of chronic diseases. Vital nutrients are absent in our cells and we are lacking adequate water.

As an example, please look up the main causes for amyotrophic lateral sclerosis (ALS), or other motor-neuron conditions. The 'medical' websites tell us that malnutrition, lack of communication between the neurotransmitters are the 'possible' causes but those are not the initial causes! There is no mentioning why the neurotransmitters don't communicate, for example. We have hundreds of different 'syndromes', which put people in wheelchairs and/or on disability. All motor-neuron abnormalities and all autoimmune disorders are the consequence of dehydration, acidosis, toxicity and oxidation.

These are caused mostly because of lack of water!

Water is the medium through which these neurons communicate.

Quite simple, not rocket science.

We are getting people out of depression often with water only! People are constipated for years, even decades and as a consequence the accumulated toxins are affecting their brain functions. Often times, as soon as they are cleaned out (the result of the detox) the depression is gone and they suddenly feel better! Fake energy drinks and coffee of course deceive the brain and the body. When we don't get enough sleep, our immune system gets compromised, we feel lousy or we have discomfort and we think we need a doctor. The first pill is prescribed pushing people quickly over the 'turning point'!

A better choice would be to make some changes in our lifestyle, drink quality water, perhaps 'spoil' the body with adequate sleep.

We learned what the root causes are but now we have to figure out how to avoid them. We got a wonderful body from our maker. We can thankfully get back to a healthy state. How?

What to Do and what Not to do, that is the question!

Can we live in a way to avoid chronic illness? Yes! I can honestly say to you that it is easier to avoid chronic situations than you might think. I like simple answers as I am a practical woman so when I learned about this tool called ERW, I embraced it. After all, how many things like this do we hear about? I only know about this one! Let me know if you are aware of something better, please. So, water would be the most important 'raw material' and the main energy source, as well, to keep us healthy but here is my list of the 'stuff' you should avoid or minimize in your life if you want to have vitality and live a pain-free life.

The list might surprise you: root canals, a dead tooth, wired bra, antiperspirants, toxic relationships, prescription pills, 'chemo', radiation, CT-scans, amalgam, stress, traumas, packaged (processed) foods, chemicals, artificial stuff, preservatives, pesticides, heavy metals, processed meat, refined stuff (sugar, flour and oils) and smoking. Illegal drugs, even if they are 'legal', they might hurt you. Just because something is legal, it's not necessarily good for the body but most of us know this.

> *"I have had a number of patients with breast cancer, all of whom had root canals on the tooth related to the breast area on the associated energy meridian."*
>
> **JOHN DIAMOND**

I hope you love humour as much as I do because it is 'mandatory.' In my father's house we used to have joking-laughing game nights once a week, on Wednesday nights. This was easy and desirable with the company we had or family members, of course; it would be crazy, however, to laugh in solitude while you are on your PC, all by yourself.

When it comes to exercise, a reasonable, constant, light exercise, something fun would be my choice. You don't have to be a 'gym fanatic' to be healthy. You need to drink water, much more than you need to be an athlete.

People in general are focusing on what not to do.

I am saying that what you don't do (and *should* be doing) is ruining your health much more than the things you are doing.

A good expression would be: Mandatory requirements! Water, should be mandatory, but people - just like I did - would rather start a revolution against water than just drink it.

I don't blame anyone who is not drinking water. Water is kind of yucky and I know this comes as a surprise but this is my conclusion;

There is a very good reason why most of us don't like to drink ordinary water! There is no water available anymore that is 'recognised' by our body or friendly to us out there! Period. Or, is there? Don't be shocked, be amazed! We will investigate!

Animal fat, for example, is not our worst enemy according to my experiences. I have known thousands of healthy people who lived long healthy lives and had none of the degenerative conditions who practically lived on naturally raised animal fat. Those who say to avoid natural and go for artificial, they are our worst enemy. Stay away from artificial products. If you don't understand what they are, please learn about them. (Margarine versus good old natural butter kind of a thing.) None of these things alone will kill anyone but the totality of unnatural lifestyle and bad habits, topped by not drinking good water can and will.

Well, that is not entirely true, one 'thing' can kill all of us (no matter how wonderful we are), on its own. Electro Magnetic Waves and fog are killing us and our children. Cell towers placed near schools and houses, for example, are causing cancer in children in unprecedented numbers. God help us as I don't see how we can stop those things. Smart phones can kill people physically and/or mentally, which is why Silicon Valley parents are restricting the use of these phones in the lives of their children. (Please watch on YouTube, the commentary on *Tucker Carlson Tonight,* which was broadcasted on Fox News, on Oct 30th, 2018. It is eye opening. They call the screens 'poisons' as they know that 'digitally distracted kids' are bad news for the future of humanity. They are pushing local schools to remove these devices from the classrooms. They are really worried about the impact of this technology on their children's physical and mental health. Our dehydrated children with their weak immune system are not strong enough to handle this new danger.

"The evidence for a connection between phone use and cancer is clear and convincing. The more you use cell phones and the greater the number of years you have them, the greater the risk of brain cancer."

PROF. KJELL MILD (Biophysicist, Sweden)

EMF becomes much more dangerous when we are dehydrated. There is not adequate extracellular water to conduct these electrical waves and nothing else will help us as much as proper hydration. The average parent is not educated about this. We must wake up to this new reality. I can't forget this young mom who was sitting on the airplane beside me holding her newborn baby in her arms. There is not much room on airplanes nowadays. Yet, after me asking her nicely twice to put her smart phone away explaining the danger as much as I could, she kept playing on the phone which she was holding near the baby's brain for five hours. Frankly, I wanted to throw her off the plane! Brain cancer is the number one killer of children under age five.

"EMF toxicity is best avoided by cellular hydration."

Dr. ZACH BUSH

Are you doing "technological detoxing" regularly? We all must if we want to live. We need a break from technology like computers or cell phones. Now, with Kangen Water® as the main tool, the different types of detoxifications will be much easier. You will see why. Spending time in the forest is another way to detox from EMF. To do that, however, you need time and you need a forest nearby. While the Kangen® machine brought both the forest and the waterfall into our home at the same time, I love to get out to nature as often as I am able.

Are you drinking and eating just about anything that's offered to you? What did the serpent say to the woman? "You can eat from the tree …. You certainly will not die." (Genesis 3.4). A very similar situation we have today. We are told by advertisers: "Eat it! Take it! Drink it! Smoke it! Just swallow it and you will get better!" Does this remind you of the sweet words of the serpent?

We are very far from 'manufacturing' food for human consumption. **None of what *we* are 'making' is good for us!** Not the drinks, not the pills, not the altered, synthetic, manufactured, or genetically modified foods. We need to grow food the traditional way and let them stay organic. Simple. (Don't you think specific genetics were built into our food for 'a good reason' to match the genetics of our bodies? We have to give some credit to the one who created this Universe! Oh wow, at times 'science' can get even dumber than someone with not much schooling.

The Bible is not only a spiritual guide, it does talk a lot about how to live and to be physically healthy, as well.

*"Within the covers of the Bible
are the answers for all the
problems man faces."*

RONALD REAGAN

*"To the Bible, man will return;
and why? Because they
cannot do without it."*

MATTHEW ARNOLD

I am sure you have heard about President Reagan but maybe you don't know Matthew Arnold (1822) who was an English poet and a cultural critic. His philosophical poems demonstrate undeniable insight. It is very cool to look back in history, let's say in 200-year intervals. Old is not necessarily out of style and wrong. Modern or new is not necessarily good or desirable. We must examine things in this light.

Think of your health or body as a bank account from which you can only take out as much money as you put in or less, **never more**. We get that, yet when it comes to our bodies, we want the maximum out and we put very little in. Not much of 'spiritual food' either but that is another story! We push hard, we empty ourselves because we lack wisdom and understanding and then we blame the doctors. We can change all that, easily, just by learning about the truth and by applying small changes to our lifestyle.

Everything, the environmental contaminants, what we breathe in, all the poisons we are exposed to, toxic sugar-laden drinks, absolutely everything ends up in the blood stream. The blood is a flowing river to all the cells for nourishment and removal of acidic waste. Our blood can be either a river of life or a river of death and disease.

"For the life of every sort of flesh is its blood, because the life is in it."

LEVITICUS 17.14

High blood pressure is caused by dehydration. Every second person is on high blood pressure pills, most people are chronically dehydrated on the cellular level. The blood is 85 percent water. When the body needs water, the easiest way to draw that crucial water is from the blood. Blood is available almost everywhere in the body. When water is drawn from the blood, it naturally becomes thicker hence dangerous as it can cause strokes and heart attacks. The body was intelligently designed to avoid sudden death. The pressure is naturally raised so the blood circulation won't be affected. It is logical. The answer is not to manipulate the functioning of the body with pills but to get water back so the pressure can normalise again. This is probably why most of the people who get on the water and drink a sufficient amount will drop the high blood pressure pills within a month.

CHAPTER 7

BACK TO ORIGIN

*"One of the truest tests of integrity is,
its blunt refusal to be compromised."*

CHINUA ACHEBE

During history we compromised much more than we should for many different reasons. That, however, will never justify getting away from the truth. 'Urgent stuff' is repeatedly getting in front of what's important. This is the way the majority thinks.

This is what I call, "A trap"!

We are on the run and we don't prioritise as we should. We lost faith in what has always been the right thing to do. We are just 'vegetating' when it comes to integrity, we don't live it! We believe or pretend to believe the stories, the BS as we think we can't do better or any different. We are not well but we got used to 'the situation'. All that should stop here, right now!

Today, I would like to raise *hope* up a notch if you have nothing against this totally reckless behaviour of mine.

Hope is important! Faith is a must!

Faith is needed like never before to find balance in a very negative world.

Today is *your* Day! Why stay in a chronic condition when all these conditions are reversible? Why even get there when most of it is preventable?

Please note that the human body runs on electricity as per natural laws. We need to understand and respect these laws. We were created wonderfully. Health is a gift, which is why I have not let it be taken from me, a few times now. At least, not without a fight! Like it or not, we are electrical beings. Negative ions play a tremendous role in achieving optimum health and body balance. For only this reason, it makes sense to drink 'living', biodynamic ionized water with a negative electrical charge versus 'dead' water. What many forget or don't understand is that we have been given a free choice in everything we do. Don't blame God. Prayers can't replace water or the right lifestyle. This is exactly why the same number of believers die of cancer and heart attacks as non-believers. No religion, spirituality or anything else of that sort will help when someone is chronically dehydrated and toxic. Water is part of our physical world. Water is 'life-giving'. This is precisely why it's symbolically used over and over again in the Bible when eternal life is mentioned.

"And he showed me a river of water
of life, clear as crystal, flowing out from
the throne of God and of the Lamb."

REVELATIONS 22.1

The masses are not educated regarding health. Kids grow up these days on junk.

What they are drinking all day long, every day, is more important than what they eat! How many people realize this fact?

(Stay with this thought for a second). Are you surprised that kids today don't have a good immune system? Children are routinely immunised with chemicals 'to prevent' disease but those only do harm by destroying their natural immunity.

There are no shortcuts in life.

Are you aware of what your kids are drinking or not drinking?

Science has already discovered that everything in the universe is an expression of energy. The atom is nothing but electrical energy, there are huge spaces within the atom itself. The central part of an atom carries a positive charge. By structuring the atoms in different ways, we get different matter. All atoms have electrons with negative charge, so they have polarity. Each one of our cells is recharged by electricity, thus everything we put in our body should have life force in it. I am sure synthetic matter doesn't have life force, period. Are you sure you want to drink regular water? I call regular water GMO, because of the additives, which alter the chemical make up and the structure of it.

"Health is life energy in abundance."

"With the right kinds of energy,
every disease is curable."

JULIA H. SUN

Are you 'recharging' regularly or do you keep pressing the gas even when you are tired? I did that sometimes in the past. Not a good thing to do.

Everything that goes into our body needs to match the matrix of the cell. We need electrons. Most of today's lifestyles including our electronics are stealing electrons from our healthy cells. Any 'manipulation' done to a living matrix changes its configuration. Most cells in our body are designed to conduct electricity. There is a very close co-relevance between pH value and bioelectricity.

A huge mistake happened when some doctors started to understand contaminated water. They wrongly assumed that purified water would be better for people's health.

They based everything on the purity of water, not knowing anything about its molecular structure!

Big lessons learned after several decades.

I personally know a woman who got very ill after using 'reverse osmosis' water for years. She was an insurance client of mine and a friend for a long time. She called me a few years ago to say she was dying.

The worst part was that no one could figure out why she was so weak. She is a nurse. This seemed unbelievable to me knowing how strong and healthy she was when we met at first as opposed to when we saw each other last. I was wondering how much she was exaggerating. The phone conversation turned kind of funny as she kept asking me about her life insurance and how the benefits will be paid out. I kept changing the subject by talking about water and how Kangen Water® changed my life since we talked. How terrible! How 'unprofessional'! My heart was guiding me for sure, not my mind. Thinking back, this might have been 'the moment' when in my heart I became a 'life agent' and ceased to be a life insurance agent. Thankfully, she listened to me as she trusted me. At first, she did not want to hear about "water" at all as "they spent a lot of money on a Reverse Osmosis System five years prior". I wanted to make sure she completely understood about ERW so I visited her in Brampton, Ontario, which is 'only' 6000 km's away from our house. In about three months, after the RO system was taken out of her house and she switched to ERW, she recovered 100 percent. About five years have passed since. Her life insurance proceeds have to wait but I am sure she doesn't mind. LOL.

Because of this information, we also helped to prolong a beautiful, six-year-old dog's life. Ely's heart was failing and the vet told the owner that he couldn't do anything more for them. The dog was medicated for years and over $10,000 was spent. As soon as I heard that the dog was drinking RO water all its life, I had to mention what we learned about water. They took two gallons of our water for Ely. The very next day he jumped off the bed, which he had not done for six months. They called me crying from happiness. These stories made me learn how important natural minerals are for us. Over three years have passed since and Ely, my friend's beloved dog, is still alive.

Throughout this book, I will aim to share facts and testimonials with you from many different sources. I don't want to give you my opinion. You can form your own understanding. You don't have to listen to those who never actually tried the water either as some of them got 'an opinion', believe it or not.

The information regarding 'dead' water is not coming from me or any of us 'Kangenites'! There is a very good document you can find online by Rummi Devi Saini, in the *Publication of the International Journal of Applied Chemistry.* (IJAC) ISSN 0973-1792, Volume 13, Number 2. Rummi Devi Saini is a chemist who studied at the College Pathankot, in Punjab, India.

The Purple Wave

He states: "The importance of minerals and other constituents in drinking water is mentioned even in the 'Rig Veda', (The oldest sacred book of Hinduism), in which properties of good drinking water are described. Water should have nutritive value and required minerals, its acid-base balance should be within normal limits... Demineralised water is highly aggressive, attacks the pipes." Knowing this, one can imagine how it pulls carcinogens from the plastic bottles and all that plastic is made of. Crude oil is a carcinogen meaning cancer causing! Further he talks about the direct effects of water low in minerals.

"Low intake of magnesium, calcium, iron and sodium on health in general and on the intestinal mucous membrane as reported by the World Health Organization (WHO), is contributing to or causing blood clotting, heart muscle contractibility, lack of conducting myocardial system, muscle flexibility, hypertension, diabetes, osteoporosis, cardiovascular disease, neuro-degenerative problems, some cancers, electrolyte imbalance, metabolic acidosis, coronary heart disease, brain edema, muscle cramps, fatigue, gastric ulcers, jaundice, anemia, fractures, growth disorders and more."

Wow. This looks exactly like today's society, doesn't it?

"Conformity to a sick society is to be sick."

RICHARD J. FASTER

I am thinking - *what if all these health issues could be stopped right at this level?* Why not? It sounds logical but I also found two doctors who believe exactly this in case I sound really crazy. Both are doctors and researchers: Dr. Hidemitsu Hayashi, a heart surgeon, and Dr. Batmanghelidj have the same opinion. One from Japan, one from Iran/Europe/America and there are many more. We will talk about this a bit later.

You might ask: Why get and/or trust information from the other side of the world? This is why I do it. Do you remember the layered lies I was mentioning earlier? The 'West' at the moment is the home of layered lies. In other words, the money now is used to protect the accumulated wealth of some industries. These industries keep lying and that is confusing to most people, of course. We just have to get used to the fact that it is not about the truth or about integrity.

> **"It is only prudent never to place complete confidence in that by which we have even once been deceived."**
>
> **RENE DESCARTES**

Shouldn't we want an 'unbiased brain' when it comes to our health? I learned my lessons and I am not alone with this. There are many studies about RO water worldwide. This article is coming from investigative reporter, Frantisek Kozisek, reporting for the National Institute of Public Health in the Czech Republic. A great example of an interesting phenomenon called 'industry harassment'.

He writes: *"I can't begin to tell you how much pleasure it gives me to write this article. I will never forget being severely chastised a few years ago by a senior executive of a company that sells thousands of reverse osmosis (RO) systems per year for, 'not knowing what I'm talking about'. He informed me that my challenge to him and the industry about RO water being unhealthy was 'preposterous'. At the time of the meeting I was not equipped to fend off his accusations because I hadn't put in the research that I have now...*

The RO industry has been disseminating inaccurate information for years.

Doctors and other health care professionals have unwittingly been endorsing the 'RO water as the best drinking water' message for years, which makes the myth worse because we trust these people with our health. *I offer two sources of evidence that unequivocally reveal the fact that the water produced by RO systems is bad for your health if you drink the water over the long term. First, the American government's online health website: The bottom line of what I learned from reviewing the studies is that your body typically absorbs anywhere from six percent to thirty percent of its daily requirement of essential elements from tap water. In a world where our soil is virtually devoid of nutrients from too many crops and not enough recovery time and where diets are anything*

The Purple Wave

but healthy, it is very important to your long-term health that you ingest calcium and magnesium from drinking water."

A second website that drives a dagger into the RO industry myth that pure water is healthy, comes from the World Health Organization (WHO). **The WHO provides us with a position paper titled "The Health Risks from Drinking Demineralized Water."**

Kozisek concludes: *"The final report, published as an internal working document (WHO, 1980), concluded that, not only does completely demineralised water have unsatisfactory organoleptic properties, but it also has a definite adverse influence on the animal and human organisms."*

The potential for adverse health effects from long term consumption of demineralised water is of interest not only in countries lacking adequate fresh water but also in countries where demineralizing home water treatment systems are widely used, or demineralized bottled water is consumed.

In summary: **"Scientific testing and the best 'unbiased' brains in the world have repeatedly demonstrated that long-term consumption of demineralized (RO) water is bad for your health."**

Mostly all bottled water is RO water. These waters often have added inorganic minerals, and some people who have these RO systems are supplementing with inorganic minerals which unfortunately can't be absorbed. Wow! Do you know that for every liter of RO water made, a minimum of six liters of water are wasted? Wow, let's thank this brave reporter for the article.

"In a time of universal deceit telling the truth is a revolutionary act."

UNKNOWN

I hope that you believe it by now: 'pure' water has to be avoided!

Unfortunately, it's not only the water, which is harming us. Free radicals are everywhere in our environment. They are causing more oxidation than we can handle. This never happened before during human history. The simple fact is that we never had this much pollution. So, where are these positively charged ions coming from? The main sources of EMF pollution are cell phones, cell towers, WIFI. Other sources are: artificial light, pollution from cars and airplanes, greenhouse gas emissions, air conditioning, microwaves, everything polluted by 'civilization'. This is what we have more and more of as we are 'progressing'. Our grandfather (many are using 'grandpa' as an excuse) who lived 100 years ago and smoked and everything else, did not have this situation. Yes, in that environment they got away without a Kangen® machine. Today, things are very different for us.

Tap water is treated to death and it has a positive charge, so it is extremely oxidising. People keep telling me that in Canada we have the best water. This is a misconception we should discuss. Sidney Harris once said "When I hear somebody sigh, 'life is hard,' I am always tempted to ask, compared to what?" This is what I am tempted to ask you: Compared to what? (Sidney is an American cartoonist, born in 1933 in New York, who is known for his cartoons about science and technology.) Yes, of course we have great water compared to those who are drinking refurbished water from the Detroit River or the water in some places in Africa. This, however, is only half of the story. The other half is this: Municipalities all over Canada and the rest of the world are mandated by law to make tap water neutral or slightly alkaline. This piece of legislation was introduced to reduce pipe corrosion. The pH of water after the necessary chlorination is normally about 3.5-4.5 pH. That is acidic enough to 'eat' the pipes. The issue of corrosion had to be taken care of by mandatory alkalization, which means more chemicals were added to the water. To get the desired 7 or 7.5 pH, ammonia, ash and other 'additives' such as lye - some quite poisonous - are dumped into the city water systems.

Chlorine in itself is rat poison. Most of us will never realise it as when we get ill, this 'poisoning' will be labelled as an illness or a syndrome. When we open our tap, we are not getting H2O plus minerals only. We might call it water but really it is something quite different. The neutral or slightly alkaline pH of tap water is chemically achieved! **I call this fake**. Nothing is going to be beneficial that is fake. (What a great word that was re-introduced recently, let's use it!) And you thought that only the News on CNN can be fake.

Originally water was perfect. It did not need treatment or alteration/ manipulation of any kind. This is what Health Canada says about our tap water:

"Recent studies done on chlorinated water revealed that regular intake of tap water has been linked to the development of several forms

The Purple Wave

of cancer...chlorinated tap water is a skin irritant and can be associated with rashes like eczema....It can destroy polyunsaturated fatty acids and vitamin E in the body while generating toxins capable of free radical cellular damage. Chlorinated water destroys much of the intestinal flora, the friendly bacteria that help in the digestion of food and which protect the body from harmful pathogens. Chlorinated water contains organochlorides, which can cause mutations by altering the DNA, supress immune system function and interfere with the natural controls of cell growth". Wow. Is this acceptable to you? It doesn't sound too good to me.

Water or food, which is largely synthetic, incomplete, modified, distorted, dead and toxic, will not benefit the body. Only energy/matter with the right matrix will enter and recharge the cell engine. This is never explained to us. Are you asking questions yet? Tyler LeBaron a leading American scientist is expressing this in a different way: *"The ORP [Oxidation Reduction Potential] of the internal environment of a healthy person is always on the reductive side, below -350 mV. Therefore, with a healthy viewpoint in mind, it would make sense that the optimal drinking water is one with a negative ORP. Water with a positive ORP is reduced to a reductive ORP at the expense of consuming the electrical energy from cell membranes."* Wow, now we know what is interfering with our cellular metabolism and what is draining our energy when in fact it should energize us.

> **"Does a sick society get so used to its illness**
> **that it can't remember being well? What if**
> **the memory is too dangerous for the people**
> **who like things the way they are?"**
>
> **NEAL SHUSTERMAN**

We are polluting everything on Earth with the speed of light or faster and we have no idea how to stop.

> **"Thank God man cannot fly, and lay**
> **waste the sky as well as the Earth."**
>
> **HENRY DAVID THOREAU**

Sorry Henry, your statement is outdated but we like the point you are making. Humans, lately do fly and fly a lot in airplanes, which do pollute the sky, the waters and everything in between. Airplane traffic is only going to get worse. Flying in planes is hard on the immune system. I don't recommend flying for anyone with a history of cancer for example. On my last trip, a 50-years-old nice lady and her husband sat beside me. She already had a blood clot incident. She had no knowledge about water that absorbs and works against strokes and blood clots by 'thinning' the blood naturally. She seemed very grateful because I talked to her about the water. **The time for ERW truly arrived.** Most of the people don't know about it and Enagic® is hiring. Do you want to make a difference in the world? So many are looking for good opportunities to be volunteers to help the environment or have something to do during retirement. Why not Enagic®?

'Crying' about the environment won't help the environment. Doing something about it will. Here is your chance. Ionization at the 'source', (your tap) will absolutely abolish the need for bottled water. Eliminate plastics by having an eco-friendly lifestyle.

You can contact me if you need help or if you would like to become an *active* advocate for nature by having an extraordinary tool to achieve that goal.

CHAPTER 8

BORN TO LOVE

"Love is what we were born with.
Fear is what we learned here."

MARIANNE WILLIAMSON

et's change the subject as there is no reason to get depressed now when you are on your journey for a much healthier life. It was and still is a beautiful journey for me.

Let's talk about love, which is always uplifting. Love is another universal 'miracle' besides water. No one can deny that love has the power to change us, recharge us, make us happy. Love somehow transcends, diminishing the differences which divide us, and makes life worth living. Love can solve problems if it's real love and not selfish. We came here because GOD loved us. We are here because he still does. He always will. Life would be different if we all would love Him and his creation back. **We were born to love!**

Klara Reid

> *"There are two great days in a person's life: the day we are born and the day we discover why."*
>
> **WILLIAM BARCLAY**

Once I watched a movie with a couple who had already 'split' (they got divorced three months prior) mostly because they could never have children. The agency where they applied to find a mother who would consider them as adoptive parents suddenly contacted them. They had been chosen by a sixteen-year-old pregnant girl as possible parents. The ex-husband already 'moved on' with a girlfriend in the picture when they were called by the agency. They got really excited and decided to play the 'show' of a happy marriage in order to get the baby.

At this point, I was thinking: here we go again, another desperate family who will do anything to become parents. I've seen numerous movies like that. The reason I remember this particular movie is because this one turned out to be different. The biological mother in the movie, the pregnant girl was 'troubled'. She was in the custody of a corrections officer. The legal system couldn't find a place for her to stay where she wouldn't get in trouble. They asked the couple to take her in and they accepted this as a temporary solution (a crazy idea) only until she delivered the baby. She wasn't easy to deal with. She had never experienced unconditional love. *How sad,* I was thinking. I expected that the couple would get upset or completely reject her crazy behavior and just take the baby from her but that is not what happened. When the girl changed her mind and decided to keep her baby, the couple did not get upset. Unconditional love was poured out, probably for the first time on this child having a baby. The couple instantly became loving 'parents' and the girl started to transform. She became easier to deal with, returned the love, and quickly turned into a new person. At the end, she kept the baby and the couple rediscovered the love they had towards each other. They got busy with their publishing business and the husband dropped the girlfriend. They decided to adopt the mother, becoming 'grandparents', this way which was more appropriate anyhow, because of their age. Everything worked out, they were all happy and things looked amazing for the future. All this happened because of unconditional love. So, why tell you this story?

I see it often when people are distracted by their 'problems', they don't act lovingly. This happens to most of us. We are reasonable but 'reasonable' shouldn't be the norm. We do better when we listen to our heart. Families suffer because of mixed-up priorities. When we put love first, amazing things happen. Love is so above everything else that it can solve otherwise unsolvable problems and put things into perspective. It's amazing how love moves things. You have to experience that. Try it! We should never fear love. All we should do is 'love' and wait and see what happens. Love truly never fails. We fail when we 'forget' to love.

Love, however, is nothing without action.

I would like to invite you to consider drinking good water and providing your family with the best possible source of water, not because of fear of illnesses like cancer or any other reason but because of that love I know you feel towards your family and you should feel towards yourself. Don't worry about money or anything else. Just have faith that if **you do the right thing, things get better and they will work themselves out.** A great blessing will always come your way when you are doing what you are supposed to do.

It did work out for us and for so many I know who took a leap of faith. For things to get better, first we have to do the right thing. Another major law of the Universe. Are you bold enough to do the right thing?

"You don't love someone for their looks, or their clothes, or their fancy car, but because they sing a song only you can hear."

OSCAR WILDE

"When you look into your mother's eyes, you know that is the purest love you can find on this Earth".

MITCH ALBOM

There will be no singing of songs together or eyes to look into if we don't take care of our family. Early death of family members is painful and heart breaking. What I hate about it the most is that it destroys the family unit and creates a hole, which will stay with us until we die. Life will never be the same for those who lose their loved ones prematurely. When a loved one suffers or dies it's much worse than when we are terminally ill. Do you agree with me? If you lost someone dear to you, you probably felt this horrible feeling.

Oops, I apologise, I got lost. It's easy to get lost in love but let's return to our subject, which is water.

"Love the world as your own self, then you can truly care for all things."

LAO TZU

CHAPTER 9

DEAR STRESS, LET'S BREAK UP!

"Stress does more than make you sick. It destroys your peace, hope and dreams."

ELLEN SOMMER

You are probably thinking - *Yeah right...if getting free of stress would be that easy.* I would like to show you how you can 'break up' with stress and it is for real. It will be an important part of a very realistic project, our 'water project'.

Fear or stress, the opposite of love, (when it comes to the well being of humans) can be detrimental. Most of the time it causes trauma in us humans. We have to deal with a wide variety of stresses in life: emotional, chemical, acidic, oxidative, electrical, and physical stressors. I had lots of crazy stress in my life. We don't have to look for stress. Stress finds us because most of us are 'realistic people'. I know I am.

> ## *"Reality is the leading cause of stress among those in touch with it."*
>
> **LILY TOMLIN**

You did not see that coming! I hope you did not deny the fact that your life is stressful...if you did, you fell right into Klara's trap. Sorry, I forgot to tell you earlier that I love to tease people...it has a stress releasing effect on me.

How we react to stress or cope with it is different for each person and that is what matters! Most people know that this is what matters but please let me share with you a secret.

The 'best' way to deal with stress is being well hydrated at the cellular level.

That is how you do it. Why? You will understand it before you finish the chapter, I promise. We are told by 'experts' that our reaction to stress is the main and most important factor when it comes to it. I have a different experience.

> ## *"It's not the load that breaks you down, it's the way you carry it."*
>
> **LOU HOLTZ**

Remember this expression: 'the way you carry it!' This now has a whole new meaning for me and you might get something out of this.

Have you ever thought about dehydration as something stressful for the body? I never had.

I carried the 'load' life put on me, without water.

I was dried out and did not know it. I will call my dried-out state 'primary' stress. The consequences were devastating. After these 'experiences' (the worst nightmares of my life) dehydration is considered by me the underlying or root cause of injury from 'secondary' stresses. What I am saying is this:

Dehydration will interfere with the body's normal ability to cope with all the other stressors.

It is not easy to discover this. It took everything I have been through plus paying attention to Dr. 'Batman's' water theory to realize this simple fact.

The good news is that stress doesn't necessarily have to cause trauma or damage in the body.

The simplest way to illustrate how important hydration is to our body's resilience to stress would be a comparison to a tree. When saturated with water, the tree has flexibility. It will move, it will bend, might lose a couple of branches when faced with the 'trauma' of the wind or the storm but it will recover quickly. When the tree is dried out (dehydrated), the same storm or even less will break it, period. There will be substantial damage, guaranteed. It is one thing to cope with stress once we are well hydrated (we won't 'break') and it is another (totally different) situation when we are dry, 'lifeless' like the tree I was talking about.

Many people's moods are also greatly affected by stress. They are 'hard to live with'. They take out their frustration on others. Families get broken up because people don't know how to get rid of the stressors in their lives and especially how to manage them on a day-to-day basis.

"I am not stressed out!! The next person who says I look stressed, gets their face ripped off!!! Understand???"

UNKNOWN

Dehydration alone will prevent you from being active, aware or happy. It will deprive you of energy and make it hard for you to perform. This is huge, I think. How many people say they don't have enough energy to cope with their lives? None of them are realizing that this is actually dryness or lack of water. If only they knew how easy it is to change this situation!

Most people think they must eat to receive the essential energy they need. Yes, good food is part of the equation but energy is produced or should be produced mainly by the water we drink. Have you heard the word 'refreshing'? How does water refresh you? What or who gives that power to water? Water only works if it's living.

One of the reasons we overeat is that our brain misinterprets our body's signals. "We often think we are hungry when in reality we are thirsty" says 'Dr. Batman'. The insights I learned from him helped me realize what was going on with me during my 'dry years'.

I never used to be thirsty when I was drinking very little water. I was always hungry. When our body is not signaling thirst any longer, it doesn't mean that we are hydrated; just the opposite. We are already in big trouble. I know that this is a bit tricky but this is how it works. Now, that I drink much more water, I feel thirst every day. My body reacted to good water and I became a huge water drinker. The 'signaling' was turned back on. I am normal again, at least, in this regard. All my body signals are working again. I get sleepy at night, which I never did, I can't wait to jump out of bed in the morning which never happened before.

I am told by many that they are never thirsty. This is sad. More than sad. **This is what I call a Tragedy!**

If you never feel thirst, you can be sure that you are dehydrated.

This undetected condition, which I call dehydration, will manifest in your life in many other ways. Ways that you wish you would not know, at all. It might just stop you from being a better performer or a happier person. It might be the reason why you are not at your best, physically or academically.

> *"The tragedy of life is not death,*
> *but what we let die inside*
> *of us, while we live."*
>
> **NORMAN COUSINS**

I had numerous "incidents", very weird ones that put me in the hospital for weeks and we (myself and my family) never realised what the root cause of my 'medical' problem was. Today, after sorting all these out, I am 100 percent certain that ninety percent of everything I have been medically 'treated' for was caused by involuntary chronic dehydration. Every time I had excess emotional stress (marital issues, accidents of family members, or extreme stress at the workplace), I ended up in the hospital. My condition was labelled as angina or a panic attack or something similar. Other times the doctors were clueless.

In two instances when I suffered 'chemically induced' stress, quite serious situations occurred. The first time a very strong coffee prepared by my ex-husband put me in the hospital for six weeks. I was taken by ambulance this time as I had a very rare episode called "sense of impending doom". I was 'interviewed' by medical students for weeks in the hospital. The doctors were not sure, so I was transferred to the psychiatric department of a different hospital in another city where I spent a month under the supervision of three doctors. It was scary to say the least. The second time ingesting high amounts of mercury for five years due to eight amalgams, I got close to death, once again. Another incident happened when I had excess physical stress (I started weight lifting in the gym) and I wound up with a serious back injury, which put me out of the gym for about five years. In all these situations, I got hurt and had different symptoms (which were always labeled as illnesses), but—a huge but—dehydration was the underlying cause. I don't know how to 'stress' this strongly enough.

What I am trying to say is that a person who is well hydrated will be able to handle the stress, or sustain much less damage from it than the one who is dehydrated. Because I was chronically dehydrated, these secondary stressors caused lots of damage, which took me out of circulation! Without the knowledge I gained and the water I am drinking I could never have figured any of this out. Divine intervention definitely happened. It is not a coincidence (as nothing is) that I am the author of this book. If I think how much money was spent on my health for those treatments, I feel guilty! When I remember how much time was wasted, I feel stupid. How could I be so naïve? I had no idea, of course, at the time. So, in case you are wondering what makes me an 'expert' on dehydration, here it is.

Once you go through something yourself, you just know it.

"Do the best you can until you know better, then when you know better, do better."

MAYA ANGELOU

I never liked to wonder much about the past. I always looked ahead, towards a better future. Always.

Let's move forward, enough about me.

There is a saying: "Thousands lived without love, not one without water". Nothing is as universal as water. What do I mean by that? Well, the populous doesn't need 6,000 different waters, for the thousands of different problems - only one, the original one! The secret recipe of 'the one' is shared here, so watch out: hydrogen, oxygen and colloidal minerals. Nothing else. End of recipe. The only water we should be drinking is Nature's water, which is H_2O plus the electrolyte minerals in it.

Water brought back to 'its original state' was all I needed. How curious! I agree. ERW solved or at least helped with a dozen different health issues I had at the time. It even 'nourished' my soul. After a couple of years drinking like crazy, I have come to life in every sense of the word. The water was crucial in helping me to restore my immune system and my health. It made me stronger and much, much happier. Can depression be a sign of a dried-out mind and/or spirit? I am convinced that it can but this might be a private affair, which remains for you to find out.

Water gives us life. You can be an asparagus or a human, it will give you life. While water is still used in greenhouses, it's not used so much when it comes to humans anymore.

"The beautiful spring came; and when Nature resumes her loveliness, the human soul is apt to revive also."

HARRIET ANN JACOBS

CHAPTER 10

THE EVIDENCE IS PILING UP

"A wise man proportions his belief to the evidence."

DAVID HOME

Our bodies are made up of about 75 percent water and the body depends on this water. Every organ depends on it and there is nothing else which is controlling the body temperature, the heart rate and our blood pressure, only water. *"It's definitely essential,"* says Jim White, registered dietitian and personal trainer of Virginia Beach, Virginia and American Dietetic Association spokesman. *"What we're finding is so many people are deficient. We're seeing a huge decrease in athletic performance and fatigue that's caused by the lack of hydration."*

People are drinking coffee like water nowadays. Many live in a myth that they had some water because water is used to make their coffee. I know however that coffee is a diuretic and a stimulant. None of that is helpful for the body. Water doesn't get the same media attention as green tea, antioxidants and the latest diets. Yet, it plays a much more critical part in our daily lives. Is certain vital information supressed by the media? You be the judge…

Apparently (I heard this today), Canadians are the most dehydrated people. Looks like drinking beer and coffee just won't do it. We will investigate!

"Those who regularly drink caffeinated beverages are literally drinking themselves dry," says Dr. Carpenter, a well-respected expert in the field. So, if you are a coffee drinker, you need even more water. Who is Dr. Carpenter? He was born in Columbus, Ohio, not that long ago. Still very young, just like I am (I am not authorised to tell you his age). This naturopath is considered an authority who has been 'playing' with all kinds of ionised water for over fifteen years. He is not only a Naturopathic Doctor, but also an Acupuncturist with over twenty-five years of clinical experience. He received a Bachelor's degree in Science from Idaho State University. He also attended the University of Victoria Naturopathic School in Melbourne, Australia and the Central States College of Health Sciences in Columbus, Ohio. He believes that an educated patient is a healthier patient. He has served on several industry Boards of Directors including the International Iridology Practitioners Association. (I have special respect towards practitioners who recognize Iridology.) He is also the author of the book called "Change Your Water, Change Your Life"!

Dr. Carpenter learned about Kangen Water® when he went to Japan to learn acupuncture. Japanese doctors were using low pH acid water to treat skin conditions including psoriasis, bed sores, diabetic ulcers and gangrene. Yes gangrene. They also had their patients drink Kangen Water® for many different health conditions. Since doctors achieved consistently impressive results in Japan, when Dr. Carpenter returned to the U.S., he began to search for a device that would produce this 'healing' water. (Kangen Water® wasn't available in North America at the time.)

He purchased a number of water ionizers and tested them by giving his patients water from these devices. His patients reported minimal improvements, if any, when they consumed the water. No device produced the results that were achieved in Japan.

It became clear to him that devices available in the U.S. simply did not produce really restructured or so-called hexagonal water. This situation never changed.

"It's not the lie that bothers me. It's the insult to my intelligence that I find offensive!"

KLARA REID AND MANY OTHERS

'Restructuring' requires power [230 Watts], which other ionisers just don't have. These machines are only 'faking it'. "Green food supplement powders could not stay in suspension", says Dr. Carpenter, "and that is one way I've come to learn to determine if hexagonal water is present in reasonable quantity." In addition, none of the devices could produce 2.5pH acidic water, which was used for treating skin conditions in Japan. When Enagic®'s Leveluk SD501® from Osaka became available, Dr. Carpenter was thrilled: "When I put my green food supplement powder in Kangen Water® for the first time and shook it up, it stayed in suspension and didn't fall to the bottom of the glass. No matter how long the glass sat on my desk, the powder didn't sink to the bottom. I knew I had found something special and what I had been searching for." He explains, "I started seeing miracles happen with my patients. This water was special. Maybe on paper other machines appear to be equal but the proof is in getting results."

Here it is, dear friends. **Different machines might appear to be equal on paper or online advertising but the proof is in getting real results, significant results.**

Make sure that you don't try Kangen Water® and then buy another ioniser. You won't have the same results. It is just a fact many will testify about. I find Dr. Carpenter's testimony fabulous but let's get back to reality in North America and Europe without this 'magical water'.

"You are not entitled to your opinion.
You are entitled to your informed opinion!
No one is entitled to be ignorant!"

HARLAN ELLISON

The truth is that the body's need for water is partially, if not completely, overlooked. I learned on my own skin that water cannot be ignored if you want to experience vibrant health. This is what I see, when I look into the eyes of society today. People have a hard time smiling or even looking into my eyes. They look lifeless to me. Their 'behavior' is very different from those who lived only 80 years ago. During the war people marching towards death had more 'life' in them than most people do these days. Do you know what is going on? Enthusiasm, real zest to life is gone or very rare. It's not normal to be alive in 2019! Do you see it? Have you noticed the 'zombie generation' yet?

Are we reflecting the *'destruction of water'*, which is grossly compromised? Some scientists say that we do.

Why are we suddenly so depressed? We will look for answers as we investigate further... I just have to catch my breath as these are serious allegations.

"There are times when we stop,
we sit still. We listen, and breezes from
a whole other world begin to whisper."

JAMES CARROL

Let's catch this new breeze together.

So, why no more emphasis on water? The answer is obvious: because water is a natural substance no one can make 'profit' on. Water can't be patented. This might be the reason why water is not recommended by health authorities. It is very rare when someone is even asked if they drink enough water or what kind of water they are drinking. So, water was left alone but that is only on the surface. During my research, I uncovered some of water's long and amazing history.

There are people who care for the truth! This is vital information to all of us after all. There are some who are interested in things other than money. There are special souls and genuine scientists who are deeply involved in different water studies.

Our first example: **Two doctors received the Nobel Prize in chemistry for the description of water channels present in the cells**

through which only water can pass. What do they mean by "only water"? Not even beer? Did you hear this? This might be a significant discovery for us, 'Canadians'! LOL. The Royal Swedish Academy of Sciences decided to award the Nobel Prize in Chemistry for 2003 for these discoveries concerning water channels in cell membranes, giving one half of the prize to Peter Agre, for the discovery of water channels and one half of the prize to Roderick MacKinnon for structural studies on ion channels. Peter Agre is an American physician and molecular biologist, Distinguished Professor at the Johns Hopkins Bloomberg School of Public Health and Johns Hopkins School of Medicine, born in 1949. Peter calls these water channels the "plumbing system" of the cell, which they truly are. MacKinnon is a professor of Molecular Neurobiology and Biophysics at Rockefeller University. Often science is only an 'educated guess' but real science is good. Real science is real.

"Science is organised knowledge..."

UNKNOWN

Another scientist who devoted his life to water and has to be mentioned is Mu Shik Jhon, from Korea. His book, "The Water Puzzle and the Hexagonal Key " is fascinating. He did enormous amounts of special tests to provide scientific evidence about how structured or hexagonal water has many different positive influences on health. Some are still ignoring his tremendous work. Mu Shik Jhon (1932-2004) was considered the world's leading authority in water science. He did forty years of scientific research. He had a B.Sc., in Chemistry, from Seoul National University, Korea (1954), a M.Sc., in Chemistry, from Seoul National University (1958) and to top that a Ph.D., in Chemistry from The University of Utah (1966). He stated: **"Aging is a loss of Hexagonal water from organs, tissues and cells, and an overall decrease in total body water. Replenishing the Hexagonal water in our bodies can and will increase vitality, slow the aging process and prevent disease."**

Really? How? Dr. Corinne Allen says: "Water is just 'smart', it knows what to do". I have to agree 100 percent. I love her natural, simple and logical approach to things. We will learn about Dr. Allen, who she is and what she does a bit later.

Dr. Mu Shik Jhon officially presented his theory on Molecular Water Environment in 1986.

That was thirty-three years ago and our North American culture is not enlightened about these findings. No wonder, we are in the dark...

"Science makes people reach selflessly
for truth and objectivity; it teaches people
to accept reality with wonder and admiration."

LISE MEITNER

Beautiful thoughts about real science.

Everything is simple, beautiful and closer to the truth if no politics are mixed in it. This is true about our water, as well.

I have my own opinion about water and this might be a bit too much for you to handle, but here it is:

"Water is more than 'scientific'.
It is divine."

KLARA REID

What is 'divine'? According to the Merriam-Webster dictionary, divine means "proceeding directly from God." I am happy with that definition. I trust Jehovah. Who is He? By the same dictionary, "GOD is the perfect being in power, wisdom, and goodness, worshipped as Creator and Ruler of the Universe". I thought it is important to mention His personal name as well, as it looks like He is definitely 'connected' to water.

Just like everything else, water was created perfect and it was meant as fuel and medicine, all in one, for all living. Science discovered that natural food and nature's water are also a source of Information. Yes, they contain information for the cells. This is why genetically modified 'foods' are so detrimental for us. They don't have the right information so our body won't recognize it and won't be nourished with it. What happened to this perfect fuel? This is what you need to know and this book might just help you!

According to scientists, who are not mainstream, we humans have destroyed the structure (the essence) of water during our crazy history. The many wars, explosives, 100 brainless years of industrialization and now the aggressive agriculture, the use of pesticides, chemicals, air traffic, ...etc., all contributed to it.

Now, please listen. Some brilliant minds have 'restructured' the water! They fixed it! How? It was as unbelievable to me as it might sound to you. It took many decades of research and hard work but it finally happened! You need this information and you need to understand why Kangen Water® will help you. Without a bit of education, this might seem a scam or completely unbelievable. However, you understand that the smart phones we have today would never have been believed 60 years ago when I was born, either. Only 120 years ago no one would have believed that airplanes could exist, let alone lift off the ground and fly. Since then, we have been to the Moon and back. Thank God for true visionaries who solve serious problems and make life on this Earth better. I am grateful for all the good we can get as we have plenty of bad happening. Am I right?

Water was overlooked by me and yet nothing else helped. I visited dozens of medical professionals, with no significant results.

By 'piling up some evidence', my purpose is to educate and not to convince anyone. The skeptics and those who have a mindset focused on how not to do things, how not to get helped or how not to find solutions, will be dismissed at the end of this chapter. I will tell you all about this amazing discovery, soon after they are gone.

If you ask me, I don't think the skepticism argument is valid. I think not learning about new, healthy ideas and solutions is laziness more than anything else. It's doing the same old, same old and avoiding the problem. Skeptics have an excuse only when it comes to doing the right thing ... because they don't object to anything in general that is sold to them at the store, or at the doctors office. They buy into anything, no questions asked. They will only argue when something truly valuable comes into question to dispute how that will never work.

> *"Water is two parts hydrogen and one part oxygen. What if someone says; Well, that's not how I choose to think about water! All we can do is appeal to scientific values. And if he doesn't share those values, the 'conversation' is over. If someone doesn't value evidence, what evidence are you going to provide, to prove that they should value it? If someone doesn't value logic, what logical argument could you provide to show the importance of logic?"*

SAM HARRIS

Oh, Sam, I will be forever grateful. I would not be able to come up with this perfect phrase, not in a million years and I needed this to formulate an answer to those who will never believe anything except that there is nothing out there worth any attention. They *do definitely believe* that. So, in a weird way, they are also believers, aren't they? Ye!.... Together, by joining forces we just scored against the skeptics and that was Fun. Thank you, Sam.

CHAPTER 11

THE LIGHT

"May it be a light to you in dark places
when all other lights go out."

J.R.R. TOLKIEN

Okay, now that we successfully got rid of the skeptic who probably picked up this book by mistake, finally we are approaching the 'light'. I hate to be in the dark in every sense of the word. Don't you?

In today's polluted world, one of the biggest issues we have to learn to deal with is Toxicity. Deficiency and toxicity- this 'medical grade' water helped me with both as soon as I gave it a try and I started drinking enough of it.

We really needed a new tool, the situation is that serious. Prayers were answered. We did receive the ultimate tool.

I welcomed 'the light', all the knowledge and wisdom, which came with this water. Learning a lot in seven years, I connected the dots. I paid attention to Nobel Prizes and new, worthy discoveries. I followed the instructions of doctors like Dr. Batmanghelidj, a very special person to my heart. I trusted my body and my body trusted the water. I don't trust allopathic medicine (modern scientific systems of medicine) when it comes to prevention and preserving health.

Water is the most simple and fascinating thing I have ever dealt with. Once we learn about these 'hidden treasures' like water, it's impossible to forget them. I am super excited. My desire is to tell everyone about them.

Having ignored water since the beginning of the industrial age, man has created over 100,000 unnatural chemical compounds, which are now everywhere going through us, just like "nature goes through us." Most of the people don't pay any attention to these things that are affecting our lives in the biggest way. They are complaining but doing nothing or very little to solve the problem.

People are busy with work and themselves or distracted with toys and celebrations - a major trap of modern society. I cut time off distractions and looked into some valuable books. I listened and attended seminars. I talked to competent people. This accumulated knowledge largely remains untold as I never have time to tell the full story to people who also never have time to listen to the whole story.

As far as I know, no one else is educating the masses about proper hydration and the truth about water quality, except us, the 'Enagic family.' We all have our specific way of sharing our special experiences. My story ended up in this book.

> **"Teaching is only demonstrating that it is possible. Learning is making it possible for yourself."**
>
> **PAOLO COELHO**

So, buckle up and be prepared to be disturbed (I was stunned by this information). A Hungarian noble man, who was a biochemist, had an extraordinary discovery. He discovered what we call 'Vitamin C' today. This is what he is known for but there is much more here. Albert Szent-Gyorgyi (1893-1986) who received a Nobel Prize, together with other great thinkers realised that **the reason that biologists stumble to this day in their understanding of living systems is that they are focused**

The Purple Wave

on *solid matter and not the cell water* where all the chemical reactions take place.

This seemed more than interesting to me. I followed this lead and things started to change. As soon as I started to focus on water quality and water intake, not the pain or the food I was eating, things shifted.

He, Szent-Gyorgyi, has maintained all his life that:

"All biological functions consist of the building and destruction of water structures and that water is the main part of the living matrix, not merely its medium." Wow, this is important! He stated that:

"The Molecular Structure of the water is "The Essence" of Life. The person who will change that structure in the living systems will change the world".

ALBERT SZENT-GYORGYI

So, it is not only water by itself but the structure of water that is considered to be the essence of life as per Szent-Gyorgyi. Why did he say that? I believe that this brilliant mind realized that one needs water with the right structure to penetrate the cell membrane to transport the nutrients into the cells where they can be utilised. He also knew that structure means functionality.

Wow, I consider this an amazing prophecy, which was fulfilled and I know who did it and when. Did you hear about it? If yes, is it implemented in your lifestyle? If not yet, please listen as this is the essence of this book. This is why we can create a better life for human kind, with Kangen Water®. We have to talk about this. So, can structure be fixed?

All of this started in the 50s. Russian and German scientists worked continuously on this for decades. They wanted to recreate nature's water, just like Dr. Coanda, in a lab, as the industrial era had affected water quality like never before. They did tons of research but did not get close enough to actually materialise the idea. They could not recreate the original structure.

The Japanese, the masters of modern technology, finally did it. It didn't happen yesterday either, but in 1965! Wow.

Why didn't it help anyone in North America and the world? Because no one knew about it! This is my point ... let's change that! We need this water in every home, much more than we need smart phones and many other things. When I learned about this technology I was hooked.

Isn't this the best news ever? To me it was and still is.

Before getting on this water I did not know that I was dehydrated or what proper hydration was in the first place. I had no idea what lack of water can cause, neither did my doctors. I wish that at least one of the many I visited had known, as for years they could not figure out why I couldn't breathe properly or what was wrong with my lungs. It took me over forty years to get the answer. After drinking Kangen Water® for three years, I was told by a specialist in Bio-energy healing, Dr. Siu that: "my lungs are only 50 percent hydrated". Dr. Martin Siu is practicing in Brampton, Ontario and he is a Traditional Chinese Medicine Practitioner. Born in Guangdong, China, he is practicing TCM for forty-eight years. He conducts seminars in 'Auricular Medicine' both in the U.S.A. and Canada.

You can imagine how dehydrated I was before if it took me three years to get to 50 percent of lung hydration capacity. We have a family history of asthma so I take the breathing issue seriously. Most asthma is caused or is made worse by dehydration. I wasn't surprised because our lungs are about 85 percent water. There is more! "Asthma and allergies are indicators that the body has resorted to an increase in production of the neurotransmitter, histamine, the sensor regulator of water metabolism and its distribution in the body...It has been shown in animal models, that histamine production decreases with an increase in daily water intake!" says Dr. Batmanghelidj. We can't correct dehydration by overdrinking at one time, water intake has to be constant!

Things add up when you really look into it. Many in Europe still wrongly believe that bottled 'mineral water' is a healthy choice. I formerly 'hydrated' myself with it when I was really thirsty. I hated regular tap water after I suffered a very bad inflammation of the liver (Hepatitis A) from poor quality water at age twelve. I was sent as an exchange student to Bucharest where the quality of water wasn't nearly as good as back in my home town, in the middle of the Carpathians. Avoiding water for years (mostly unconsciously of course), I became so dehydrated that at age twenty when a surgeon was attempting to take my appendix out, he had to 'look' for it as it was so shriveled up and dried out. Finally, he scraped it off my kidney or what was left of it, anyway. I realized this as I have never forgotten what the surgeon told me following the surgery.

The Purple Wave

I recognized the symptoms I used to have, documented in Dr. Batman's book as "false appendicitis pain". Is this funny or sad?

Our body is an amazing machine. It will always take water from where it is needed the least and will bring it to where there is a vital need for it. I trust my body's 'intelligence' a zillion times more than I trust pills. We should listen to our body before we engage in the next diet trend or a 'fake treatment' method. We must consider being our own 'doctor' if we want control over our health. Most of what I know is because I lived it, felt it, experienced it. Dehydration, you see, is cumulative. The biggest problem is that once the brain is affected, it won't tell you that you are thirsty. Most people don't feel it when they are dehydrated; instead, they just 'pull a muscle' and they think that's just how it is. People die of stress and have no idea that the same stress would not cause death or harm, if they were properly hydrated.

> **"The idea is to die young as late as possible."**
>
> **ASHLEY MONTAGU**

I will never forget the famous Russian athlete and Olympic skater and how he died of a 'heart attack'. Sergei Grinkov, in case you don't remember this incident, which at the time shook the athletic world, was the skating partner and husband of the sensational pair skater Ekaterina Gordeeva. He collapsed and died in November 1995 at a Lake Placid arena in New York, at age 28.

After being 'fit and healthy' all his life with absolutely no signs of any illness, his death was caused by physical stress and prolonged dehydration. This was the root cause of his 'undetected' high blood pressure, which killed him. His death could have been easily prevented by paying attention to hydration.

> **"The death of a young person for no reason, is an apocalypse."**
>
> **DAVE EGGERS**

It is easy to get dehydrated when you are such an athlete as you sweat a lot. Drugs and/or steroids were ruled out in his case. How tragic. Dr. Batmanghelidj explains it very clearly, how High Blood Pressure is really a 'dehydration state'. This simple thing is a secret kept from most people. The falsehood of marketed drinks is destroying athletes like never before. The blood is slightly more than 80% water.

"The concentration of the blood can be altered by excess drinking (increases water content), excess sweating (decreases water content)"- this is from a medical site. Now you see how dehydration (high blood pressure) happens in the case of excess sweating. How simple. Athletes are not educated nor will an average doctor or coach ever explain this to them. In my opinion, this is why Sergei Grinkov died.

Lately we hear more and more about people accumulating water in their lungs. Why does the body do that? The only logical explanation I have heard is coming from Dr. Batmanghelidj. The body goes into panic mode because it is lacking water so it starts retaining it. It is a kind of self-preservation. This is exactly what happened to a friend who recovered beautifully from diabetic gangrene when he purchased a Kangen® machine. He almost lost his leg prior to drinking the water. He had many different stressors as he was on multiple pills for blood pressure and other issues. He functioned very well for about three years. The water helped his kidney get rid of the toxins from the meds he was taking. He really benefited from ERW. Then, they took a longer vacation and his water wasn't available to him. His health was fragile, of course. His lungs started retaining water and he developed pneumonia. He recovered in the hospital but it was a difficult situation. Now he is off the water as he was advised not to drink it. This is very bad news for him and his diabetes. I am worried about him. Now you understand why we travel with our Kangen® machine.

I am not trying to be smarter than the health care providers, all I am saying is that we are contributing to these situations, we are risking our health because of our ignorance. In my opinion, it is not very smart to wait until our body goes into panic mode. It is kind of late to start digging the well when we are thirsty, isn't it? Most people, including physicians, don't understand that these things are connected.

A couple of times, I've had strange episodes labelled as a 'panic attack' and I know that the lack of water was a major contributing factor if not the main cause of it. A business partner of mine had several of these panic attacks and twenty years of allergies with a couple of incidents of anaphylactic attacks but not one since she started drinking Kangen Water®. Five years have passed. No one will make me believe that this is a 'coincidence' and neither are the many different cases I witnessed.

Good quality water will be accepted by your body! If you are not liking the water, the reason is the low quality of the water you are drinking.

We have a neighbour who has a small dog. Every day when they are walking by, this dog is looking for Sky's water, ever since we gave him some two years ago. The owner keeps pulling him away and tells us that she just gave him water. A smart dog, what can I say? The truth is, Kangen Water® is unforgettable!

*"Nothing is softer or more flexible
than water, yet nothing can resist it."*

LAO TZU

Nothing and no one. Isn't that the truth? Those who do resist it will definitely pay the price as I did.

CHAPTER 12

NUMBER ONE

*"We forget that the water cycle
and the life cycle are one."*

J.Y. COUSTEAU

G rasp this marvellous truth! *"The water cycle and the life cycle are one."* Think about this for a moment. Meditate on it if you have to...

Are we looking for the root causes or we are satisfied with the answer or the diagnosis? – "It was a heart attack" or "It was cancer"!? We have to go further than that! – I hope you do, too!

The day is not long enough for me to tell you what other problems dehydration has caused me. It affected most of my adult life and almost killed my child at birth causing a stroke to her. My beautiful daughter, Eleonora, was so 'thirsty' that she came one month early. Not only did I avoid water during pregnancy but I lost tons of water from vomiting almost every day for eight months before she was born and another five months after her birth. This would be the main cause of the inexplicable phenomenon of premature birth? - I am thinking. I must be going crazy! I am not a doctor; I am a simple woman and I do not want to make big discoveries. Honestly. Guess what? I was told by a doctor in Romania that the reason why I have pain and I am vomiting almost continuously, if I eat anything at all, is because my stomach was 'dislocated' by the pregnancy. Forty years later, this is what I have found: "You often come across the classic dyspeptic pain called Hiatus Hernia, which means displacement of the upper part of the stomach through the gap of the diaphragm into the chest cavity. This would be an unnatural place for the stomach to be. With the part of the stomach in the chest, food digestion becomes painful.**....** **Dyspeptic pain, no matter what other pathological label is attached to it, should be treated by regular intake of water."** Dr. Batmanghelidj comments on this further;

"The current use of meds is not to the benefit of a chronically dehydrated person whose body has resorted to crying for water."

Yes, indeed my body was crying for water for thirteen months and I did not know it. So, the underlying cause for my misery once again was dehydration. This makes so much sense. The nightmare wasn't over. There was more damage; extreme thirst affected my baby, as well. She came one month early and suffered a 'stroke', which affected slightly the motoric nerves in her brain. Thankfully she did not get paralysed as our amazing pediatrician, who had just got into the clinic, realized what was going on and kept her under oxygen for five hours, until her breathing normalized.

Another thing I learned from my favorite book is that morning sickness, which was a real torture for me at the time, was also because of dehydration. Throwing up made me even more dehydrated. I entered into a vicious cycle. I wish I knew it then. This is what Dr. Batmanghelidj is saying about angina pain, which I also had for over ten years which was 'treated' by nitroglycerin. "In summary: Dyspeptic pain is a thirst signal associated with chronic or severe dehydration in the human body. It can also coexist in conjunction with other 'thirst pains', like angina." Damn it, I had those two "coexisting" pains and it was scary at the time. I was so young. I wondered a lot: why is this happening to me? Angina attacks are not fun. I feared death at times and the thought that my kids will be orphans was driving me crazy.

What I find absolutely mind-blowing is that even well-meaning, eminent doctors know very little about dehydration or it is not even a consideration to mention it.

Most dieticians and nutritionists, even some Natural Health Practitioners have never heard about the number one nutrient: Water!

Proper and permanent cellular hydration, tragically, remains unknown to many. Just as we change the water in the aquarium to keep the fish alive, we should be cleaning our cells constantly by changing our water, providing our cells with vital Oxygen.

Most symptoms, which are called 'allergies' actually clear up once our cell water is 'clean'.

Eighty percent of babies today are born with severe allergies because of the tainted body fluids of the mothers.

Think about that. If we think of our body being a fish tank (which it is) perhaps then we won't neglect to clean our cells regularly. Hopefully we won't forget this analogy; none of us want the 'fish' to die!

Let's examine another aspect of wellbeing and vitality. I hope you know more about bowel management than the average person. It is an important habit to stay healthy. We clean our house, our garage, even our driveway, but we are ignorant when it comes to gastro-intestinal cleansing.

> *"In understanding the basics of digestion,*
> *you'll discover who is in charge.*
> *Here's a hint. It's not you."*
>
> **NANCY MURE**

The world-famous Bernard Jensen (1915-2008) writes, *"Autointoxication is currently the number one source of misery and decay we are witnessing in society today."* Some people carry kilograms of toxic matter inside the colon. Detoxification is often neglected and underestimated in the healing arts despite the fact that all health professionals realize that a sick body is a toxic body.

"When digestion becomes poor, we must deal with insufficient absorption of nutrients", says Dr. Jensen. He was another giant in medicine from California but you won't hear about him much in medical circles. He stated and maintained his opinion all his long life (93 years) that: "Death begins in the colon!" He was initially a chiropractor and a fantastic nutritionist, an internationally leading holistic healer who was an expert in tissue cleansing. He was running multiple health sanatoriums

The Purple Wave

and personally treated over 350,000 patients. He promoted Iridology, discovered by another Hungarian man, with the name Ignatz Peczely (1826-1911) who was a physician and a graduate from the eminent University of Vienna.

It is quite a story how this doctor discovered Iridology. As a child, he accidentally broke an owl's leg. He observed that a black line formed in the owl's lower iris at the time of the injury. After the owl's leg healed, the young Peczely noted that the black line had changed appearance. Much later, as a physician, he treated a patient with a broken leg in whose eyes he observed the same black spot at the same location. Intrigued by the possibility of a connection between physical ailments and eye markings, observing his patients, he became convinced of a connection. In 1881, he published his theories in a book called: *"Discoveries in the Field of Natural Science and Medicine: Instruction in the Study of Diagnosis from the Eye"*. This revelation prompted Dr. Peczely to draw the first iridology chart. I consider Iridology a safe and important way to tell if the body is dealing with issues and what they are without expensive or invasive testing.

Think about how our health care would look with all the doctors practicing like him?

How much money would be saved if this modality of health care would be popular today?

He also taught hundreds of other practitioners; I personally know one of them. She is an amazing woman; her name is Betsy Vouratoni. She is the best Iridologist I know. She was the healer in Toronto who helped me to open my eyes – so to speak. Why are we sweeping so much knowledge and history under the rug? Why aren't these discoveries part of our everyday life and medical therapies? This has to change!

> *"He who has health has hope;*
> *and he who has hope has everything."*
>
> **ARAB PROVERB**

Dr. Jensen taught a lot about achieving balance between spiritual, mental and physical health. These are much more connected than people can imagine. What is it, if not water, which brings the three 'dimensions' together, I am thinking? How can water do that? This is one of the mysteries we are trying to solve. The ancient Greeks already knew that in order to have a healthy spirit one needs a healthy body. Dr. Jensen is the ultimate definition of a true holistic practitioner. He published 50 books, received global awards and became a truly historical figure. He should never be forgotten. He brought Iridology to a new level. So, what is Iridology? A totally non-invasive but real and accurate diagnostic testing through the careful analysis of the iris. An Iridology test was done on my son and that probably saved his life. At doctors' regular check ups, year after year, we were told that he is fine, ok, 100 percent, healthy, etc. Other than low energy and a "learning disability" there were no other symptoms. Betsy however saw huge dark "holes" in his iris and expressed concerns. He appeared to be "near to a cancerous stage". I took this warning very seriously. I know it in my heart that my son would not be alive or healthy today if we did not do a 100 percent change in his diet. Now, approaching forty, he is a strong, healthy man and an exceptional locksmith, intelligent and smart, a Kangen Water® drinker, of course. Previously to drinking water, he was suggested to go on meds permanently for "vertigo" by a doctor. It turned out he was grossly dehydrated. Today he is successful in life. At age eighteen, he was an absolute 'vegetable'. Thank you, Betsy and thank you, Enagic®! It is extremely painful to be the parent of a mentally or physically ill child. The good news is that we can change that. Totally.

I used colonics done by a professional for years as it helped me to detox when I was so ill. Now, get this; since I started drinking Kangen Water®, I have no accumulation of toxic waste in my colon. I was looked at many times before and twice after. *"Proper bowel management doesn't require a bowel expert. One must be aware of 'the laws' of the body and follow them,"* says Dr. Jensen, this amazing healer. The "law" here means: adequate water! People with a colon full of garbage or toxic waste are given pills, not water. How would you like to wash your dirty dishes with magic pills? I prefer water.

"I do not suffer from insanity.
I enjoy every minute of it."

EDGAR ALLEN POE

The Purple Wave

Dehydrated people are given a 'water pill', which dehydrates them even more. **Insanity squared.**

Dr. Ralph Cinque says: *"Diuretics constitute a medical mischief that has to stop."* Yes, it should stop but the opposite is happening. We see more and more people falling for water pills. When you take a water pill, the result is 'pharmaceutical dehydration'. It doesn't address the real cause and it doesn't normalize anything. Dr. Ralph Cinque is a retired chiropractor born and raised in New York City. He studied in Portland, Oregon at Western States Chiropractic College. He is well known for being one of the most experienced fasting practitioners in the world. For many years, he operated the Hygeia Health Retreat in Yorktown, Texas. People came to his fasting retreat to lose weight, overcome bad habits and addictions.

The Journal of the American Medical Association (JAMA) is a peer reviewed medical journal. It publishes original research, reviews and editorials covering all aspects of biomedical sciences. In 2002, they reported that patients with kidney failure who were using diuretics had a 70 percent higher death rate than those who did not. Think about that!

"Statistics are like a bikini.
What they reveal is interesting.
But what they hide is vital."

AARON LEVENTEIN

The most trusted natural diagnosing methods in my humble opinion are Iridology and Live Blood analysis, simply because the blood and the eyes don't lie. They will also show the root of the problems. They are not catering to 'sickness labels', which really have no way of telling what should be done to rectify the problem. The blood test done by these experts, (one drop only) will show accumulation of mucus, yeast, parasites and other stuff which won't be revealed by CT-scans, not even by the many tubes of blood from a regular lab. These revelations are very important as excess mucus in the body will lead to the starvation of the cells, and cancer for example. These helped me more than all the expensive testing done at conventional labs and hospitals. There are some good specialists out there who can help you. Unfortunately, they are not covered by mainstream medical and government plans but they are well worth your money.

I know quite a lot of people who are diet fanatics and they don't pay any attention to water. I did lots of informal surveys in the last six years. It is shocking how many people ignore water altogether.

It took me ten months or so to get back into the habit of drinking enough water. Some people drink water but have no idea that only ten to eighteen percent of regular tap or bottled water is absorbed into the cells, the rest just goes through them. Why is that? We will investigate... It is unfortunate, but regular or bulk water is compromised. It travels in pipes for hundreds of miles and is bombarded with additives because of the pathogens in it. It is only good for washing dishes and flushing the toilet. I do not cook with tap water. I don't even cook with bottled water. This is why: According to the Natural Resources Defense Council (NRDC) report, Swimming in Sewage (Feb 2004): **"AQUAFINA uses the Detroit River as one of its main water sources," and, "33% of bottled water tested contained such a high level of synthetic chemicals, bacteria and arsenic that they violated industry standards."**

According to the American Journal of Nursing (November 2005): "900 deaths and 900,000 reported cases of illnesses are attributed to tainted water annually". I am wondering about the unreported number! I believe that you will help anyone, especially your loved ones if you give them this book or talk to them about the issue of drinking water. It will take a lot to get the message out but I am not giving up any time soon. I am certain that there are millions suffering who can be helped by this information. We however have to value even these compromised sources of water, as we need this water in order to make Kangen Water®. The Kangen machine won't produce water from nothing. It will bring the water back into it's natural state. That is all what it does, and that is a lot.

"Learn to light the candle in the darkest moments of someone's life. Be the light, that helps others see; it is what gives life its deepest significance."

ROY T. BENNETT

The Purple Wave

Besides drinking water, we also need to talk about the water we use for cooking. All my family members who I learned from have been very clean in the kitchen meaning that they were cooking clean food. Today we have such a scary situation with chemicals like never before. We also have many cases of food contamination that are not reported on the news any more because they are so common.

We have carcinogens like pesticides, fungicides and other horrible stuff sprayed on our food. I know that most of the people don't realize this as they have never been told, however that won't change the fact that these are poisons. If you don't prepare clean food for your family, it is better if you don't cook, at all. It is not the end of the world; you can always turn your kitchen into an extra bedroom, perhaps into a social media room? Don't forget however that poisons will make you toxic, toxins will cause acidosis and acidosis is the right terrain (environment) for cancer.

CHAPTER 13

THERE IS A WAY

"Every discomfort and uneasiness around your chest and heart is not because of relationships and love. Sometimes it could be because of acidity."

THE UNKNOWN WRITER

We live in an acidic world and that is a fact. How acidic? You do the math. Rain water normally is around 5.6 pH. It used to be around 6.2-6.3 pH. What they measured in the USA in 2000, however, was 4.3 pH Acid Rain. Acid rain is also common in southeastern Canada.

Measurements carried out in two industrial cities on the northern and northeastern Tibetan Plateau demonstrate how fast human activities have been increasing rainwater acidity. In a period of thirteen years the rainfall pH value in the city of Germ has dropped from 8.03 to 6.8, representing a manifold increase of the H+ concentration.

Six is 100 times (10 x 10) more acidic than eight on this scale, rather than the difference of two. (The pH scale is logarithmic, meaning the value between the numbers is not one but tenfold.) **Drinking fluid that is**

100,000 times more acidic than your blood pH is crazy and down-right dangerous. That equals the acidity of battery acid.

In order to keep the blood within normal range (pH 7.365-7.4) to avoid death or coma, the body has to work 100,000 times harder in the event you are drinking carbonated drinks (2.5-3 pH). All that acid has to be neutralised and that process takes tons of minerals from your body. **The tiny difference of 0.1 in the fluctuation of the blood pH makes a difference of 60 percent more oxygen in the blood.** Think about this before you buy something like that. A Live Blood analysis allows you to see how structured water can change the blood. It made it easy for me to understand why I was sick when I had my blood cells stuck together in a formation, which in the medical world is called a 'rouleau'.

The reason why the 'water-cure' works (and we know it does) is that lack of water or cellular dehydration is simply the root cause of the problem- so getting water back into the cells is obviously the solution.

We are not 80 percent chemicals but 80 percent water at birth!

Without adequate water there is no effective way of flushing out the toxins from the cells and there is no cleaning of the digestive track. There is a phenomenal and easy way to get rid of acid waste and to alkalize and hydrate the body at the same time. That is by drinking Kangen Water®, or in its scientific term, ERW.

The minerals we need so badly are present in Kangen Water®.

The Kangen® machine is not a filter, it is a Certified Medical Device, certified by the Ministry of Labor and Welfare of the Government of Japan. The water, however, before it goes through the special process called 'ionisation' or electrolysis it gets filtered for obvious reasons by a special carbon filter that is quite sophisticated, as it removes the chlorine and additives without taking the essential minerals from the water. Through this process we get ERW or restructured hexagonal water, also called small water. One of the results of electrolysis is that the ion-making minerals, like calcium and magnesium, iron and potassium are separated from the ion-breaking minerals such as fluoride, for example. This is possible, because of the naturally occurring 'ionic charge' of metals and minerals. (Fluoride is horrible for your health contrary to massive propaganda by some dentists and even medical doctors) This way we create great-tasting, naturally alkalized water. This is the only water, as far as I know, which has the power to *alkalize* the body. These essential minerals are not replaceable by inorganic minerals and they are unequivocally essential for human health. This is like going back to the original state of the water when only pure elements were in it like oxygen and hydrogen. This water can't be made by adding baking soda or other inorganic additives therefore all commercially produced 'alkaline' waters are a scam or GMO, yet again! Period. No exceptions.

> *"Who would've guessed that by simply eliminating GMOs from my diet, I could lose twenty pounds, drop my blood pressure by forty points, and level out my blood sugar levels...all in just twenty-one days!"*
>
> **BRETT ALLEN**

Another thing I have learned during my research is that not only are we not getting enough minerals from purified waters (reverse osmosis or distilled) but we also lose precious minerals stored in our muscles and bones. Water, having memory, always aims to get back to its natural state. Acidic drinks will not leave the stomach until they pull and get the 'buffer'(minerals) to neutralise that acidity. This is precisely why the pyloric sphincter is pH sensitive and it would not open in case we are drinking acidic stuff, so it will protect the pH of the blood (at any cost). The pyloric sphincter is a strong ring of smooth muscle at the end of the pyloric canal, which lets food pass from the stomach to the duodenum. It controls the outflow of gastric contents into the duodenum.

Over-acidity leads to osteoporosis (loss of Calcium and other minerals) cancer and other serious health problems. This is quite simple but very important information everyone should know about. Most kids are absolutely amazed at schools when they hear about this from our volunteers who educate them. My husband Fred along with others is one of the volunteers who like to teach kids about the horrible health implications of marketed drinks.

Kids need to hear that when they don't take care of their body, they will become nutritionally 'bankrupt'.

It is insane how this world bought into the bottled water trend. What we are creating when we go along with this is disastrous. Why are we letting this happen? Since the day I realised the truth about bottled water, I never purchased another bottle. We saved lots of money. In my opinion if you live in a city anywhere in the world today, it is impossible to nourish yourself with healthy water unless you have a portable device like the Kangen® machine. This is another point I am trying to make. People don't know that there is a solution like the Kangen® machine to take care of this major problem once and for all. We have to get the word out.

Please watch the documentary called "Water, the Great Mystery", on YouTube. Water, as a living organism, should never be contained in a bottle especially not in poor quality plastic. It doesn't matter what it is called - Super healthy, FIJI, Oxygen water, Dasani, Hydrogen water, Alkaline Water or anything else - if it's sold in a store or a restaurant in a bottle or package, it's harmful. Period. Those who 'manufacture' water, they are only after your money and as far as I am concerned, they have no right to do what they do. Athletes are the most dehydrated. Former NFL players and others are apparently showing signs and symptoms of brain traumas and concussions. There are huge class action lawsuits, chaos, blaming the wrong people ... and the cause of the problem is not addressed. Why are they so dehydrated? This type of thing has only occurred since athletes began drinking everything but water.

These people are still very young and their life is over. I am very curious when these marketed drink companies will be brought to justice.

"Before we work on artificial intelligence, why don't we do something about natural stupidity?"

STEVE POLYAK

The truth is that water is taken from the cerebrospinal fluid, the protective layer of the skull so this can't protect them from concussions or some other kinds of brain damage. This is happening because of extreme dehydration. Here you have it! Are you concerned about a child?

$H2O$ in itself will not conduct electricity. The electrolytes (minerals) found in natural water, however are amazing conductors. (This is why ionisation of the water is possible). No wonder proper hydration is the first recommendation of scientists who are concerned about the harmful effects of EMF, generated by cell phones, cell towers and electronics in general.

Furthermore, when we exercise, our body will take from our mineral reserves to neutralize the acid (lactic acid, that is) created by physical stress. The very idea that lactic acid and the pain which comes with is a normal thing it's a myth. Growing up and skating a lot I used to have lactic acid buildup and terrible pain often (now I know it was mostly because of dehydration) no matter what kind of sports I tried. It is absolutely non existent since I am drinking Kangen Water®, no matter how much energy I put out while I exercise. We need to exercise. Now I know that lactic acid is not a normal thing which "comes with exercise". We definitely shouldn't stop exercising, get hydrated instead. Health-oriented and informed athletes (most big players internationally) now use Kangen Water®!

Many athletes, however, don't have a good water source and they are getting hurt. Unfortunately, most of them are looking to get electrolytes in all the wrong places. All energy drinks are harmful. They only provide energy for the moment and then reality kicks in. People have to deal with the consequences. A new industry has been developed to replace hips and knees because of the marketed drinks people are consuming. We did not hear about hip replacement 50 years ago! The acid deposited in the joints from lack of proper hydration and marketed drinks can cripple users in just a few years. Make sure what you are consuming is not acidic and/or acid-forming. It is quite easy to check the acidity of your water or beverage. Please use a "pH indicator", which will show the whole spectrum of the pH scale. I will let you know what a pH indicator is, soon enough. Perhaps if you see it with your own eyes, it will be easier for you to understand just how bad marketed drinks are.

I don't know about you but it is hard for me to digest the fact that we are offered the very things, which are known to ruin our health at every corner. It is shocking that absolutely no one cares and no regulations are in place regarding this in our country. Our politicians are busy with other important things like accommodating people (0.00000001 percent of the population) with separate washrooms. They are ignoring the 60 percent or the 95 percent; it doesn't matter that millions die or become disabled. No one is limiting evil, just the opposite. It is promoted every day. We live in a 'free society', after all. Free to be killed and free to kill.

Sad news ... kids actually die when they overdose on energy drinks, which is quite easy to do when you become addicted to them. What a tragedy. If you are a parent, you need to educate your kids about

The Purple Wave

these dangers. Kids only want to feel great, energised and capable. I am concerned about young dancers, as well. They also lose tons of water during dancing.

These are only some of the reasons why **Kangen Water® is a necessity, not a luxury.** It is the only attainable and safe solution I know about. Do you have a reliable source of water for your family?

"The true creator is necessity who is the mother of our inventions."

PLATO translated by Jowett

I know there is lots of criticism about the driving force of inventions being science but the best inventions, in my opinion, are coming from necessity.

Anyhow, your child doesn't need a smart phone or a tablet more than he/she needs healthy water! It has become my passion to make people aware of these things. At times I sound like a broken record. I cannot do anything about how people react when they hear something they don't want to hear. They still need to hear it! You don't stop telling your kids what's right just because they don't like to hear it…do you? It makes me mad to see families losing loved ones early in life. Previous generations got killed by wars. **We are killed 'peacefully'!**

I lost both my parents way too early. The same pain losing both his parents to cancer made Robert Wright, [director and founder of the American Anti-Cancer Institute/International Wellness Centre] conduct research all his life and look for the truth. He wrote an unbelievable book called "Killing Cancer - Not People". Bob is so dedicated to the truth about cancer that I have never come across anyone like him before. Please go to the website, www.AmericanACI.org, if you need vital information or want to donate for a real project, which will actually make a difference. Bob is everything that the Cancer Society is not! He is totally independent and non-controlled. (Non-filtered, I guess, is the better word.) I have joined Bob in his fight.

The same pain was felt by Dr. Myron Wentz when, at age seventeen, he lost his father to heart disease.

Similar pain and agony caused Dr. Shinya to dedicate his life to medicine. He lost his young wife, only one year after moving from Japan to the United States and he almost lost his children because of the drastic change the family experienced by switching to the standard American diet (SAD). He left Japan for New York to complete a surgical residency at Beth Israel Medical Center. Most of the fundamental principles of colonoscopy were developed by Dr. Shinya. His other major contribution was the invention of "electrosurgical polypectomy". Shinya instinctively thought that the polyp was the forerunner of colon cancer and that removing these polyps could reduce the risk. Dr. Shinya's primary focus from his first experiences with colonoscopy was a non-invasive method of performing polypectomy. He performed the first polypectomy in 1969. This made him very famous worldwide. According to Michael Sivak Jr. and other experts in the field, this is the most important achievement in gastrointestinal endoscopy. Dr. Shinya performs surgeries on presidents, famous stars, kings, queens and billionaires. His amazing book called "The Enzyme Factor" is a classic. In this book, he is claiming that he has "zero reoccurrence of cancer" within his patients.

I call this a real achievement.

Have you ever heard about anything like this by conventional cancer treatments? Its very interesting - but not surprising - that a physician and inventor of this magnitude is recommending and is working with Kangen Water®. More than that! He would not see the patient unless they were on Kangen Water® for a minimum of three months. Not on ionised water, not on alkaline water or any other water, but Kangen Water®. Read the book. Please don't get confused just because your physician never heard of ERW. Some are not in a hurry to catch up with marvellous discoveries, others are so busy they have never heard about it. We 'Kangenites', however, are regularly selling Kangen® devices to physicians, dentists and naturopaths and that is Good News!

The stories are real, the pain is paralysing and is affecting all of us.

"God whispers to us in our pleasures,
speaks in our consciences, but shouts
in our pains. Pain is His megaphone,
to rouse a deaf world!"

C.S. LEWIS

So true! Do you need more evidence of a Creator? It is not normal to live with pain. Painkillers, however, are fraudulent. The pain tells us that something is wrong. Pain is good. Thank GOD for pain! Age doesn't come with pain. Look up the Hunzas and you will realize why they are smiling. I think they are smiling because they have a lot to smile about. They live free of pain and chronic conditions with no pharmacies or medical plans available to them. They are water drinkers and they are happy.

I call that real freedom!

The prevention of these early and unnecessary deaths should be society's number one priority.

Unfortunately, it is not taken seriously by most. One thing I know for sure is that man-made products will never replace the natural. Synthetic estrogen and chemicals in general are destroying our lives causing hormonal issues and more. The fantastic documentary called *"The Disappearing Male"* has to be seen by your entire family. You will find answers, guaranteed. Find it on YouTube, it is free to watch, and it is better (much more interesting) than an average movie.

Water is not a dogma, a religion or a philosophy. You don't have to believe in it, you just have to drink it!

Some want to 'understand' water instead of drinking it. They are not willing to put in the time to study water, however. I think that at times, true understanding means understanding that you don't have to understand it.

You can be healthy without understanding everything that is going on in your body or the universe.

Common sense should come before 'science'. We know what is driving mainstream science today. Just like it drives everything else. Money!

Why not just accept what we know and try what we can, especially when there is no risk involved.

It's a fact that we are made of water and we run on water. It is almost guaranteed that you will be injured if you don't take hydration seriously.

Our muscles lose flexibility big time when we lack water. The brain won't work properly if is not hydrated. Once I saw a man going into a shock or a seizure of some kind at the next table in a restaurant, just from drinking soda. It was scary. When he was "revived," the waitress asked him if he had epilepsy. He did not. His brain just shut down so he kicked the table and all the dishes were flying all over the place. I personally thought that he died right there. After a while he was revived and did not know about anything that had happened. It was the weirdest thing I ever saw. We immediately realized that he was terribly dehydrated.

I came across an interesting book (I was literally drawn to it at an airport while traveling) called "Brain on Fire". The book documented a true story with the precision of a reporter. A motion picture was also made based on the book. This story is very important to me as it is the exact replica of a period of my life. I was thirty-three at the time. This is another true story besides mine, which reveals a crisis situation, crucial from our stand point, showing how dehydration can manifest in different situations. By going through this myself, I ironically know more about this than most doctors. I know that dehydration created this crisis. A young journalist, Susannah Callahan, goes through an absolute ordeal. A sudden 'crazy period' is interrupting her life, her work, and no one including her doctors can find what is causing the seizures and hallucinations. All this was new to her; she had no precedent, nor had any illnesses. Up to this point Susannah and I, we had the same experiences. In her case, however, specialists went as far as a brain biopsy, which is a three-hour surgery to find out why her brain was 'on fire'. They actually told her that her brain is on fire, but they had no idea why. They could not find the root cause and with their wrong prospective, they never will. A bit of common sense would help but her doctors had the 'complicated mind syndrome'. Why not use the 'syndrome' theory on them? They invented it, after all. Sorry, for being mean but I know what I know.

This was a combination of living on coffee (which dehydrates and robs you of all minerals, especially Magnesium!), not enough sleep (she was over-stressed), and not drinking water. She wasn't feeling good and she kept going to Starbucks for coffee. Her brain couldn't handle the crisis caused by the stress of dehydration.

*"We are all born ignorant, but one must
work hard to remain stupid."*

BENJAMIN FRANKLIN

Firefighters know what to do when something catches on fire. Brain specialists in the United States could not figure out how to help this woman. Weeks of investigation got nowhere. She had a horrible time; her parents were worried sick and no one had a clue what was going on. Because no cause was found, her condition was given a new label, which did not explain anything. Her famous specialist came up with a new label. Good for him, he is paid a lot, so he should come up with "something" at least if he could not help Susannah. Eventually she bounced back, probably because she got hydrated intravenously. The story ended with a huge question mark. Not for me. Here is the thing;

Not being able to sleep because of emotional stress and being dehydrated is an extremely dangerous combination. You start having seizures and when you are out of seizures, you start hallucinating.

How do I know this? Unfortunately, I have learned it by experience. I am ashamed to admit it, but it is true. I spent two weeks at St. Joseph Hospital in Toronto and five months drugged down and out of circulation in 1987 because of an identical episode. Thankfully, God granted me a doctor who knew what he was doing. I was tied down for a day or two, not sure for how long exactly but I remember the hallucinations I experienced as if it was yesterday. At this point, I wasn't sleeping at all, nor was I drinking much water for two weeks. Life got so crazy at home, that I couldn't. The hallucinations seemed so real and vivid that I was peeing in my bed. I was convinced that the bathroom was a gas chamber. No one could take me in there or convince me otherwise. Thank you, Dr. Jeney, for saving my life. (Dr Jeney is a Hungarian doctor in Toronto and he was just before retirement; the reason that he was called was because I could not communicate in English at the time). I am wondering how many people are put on drugs permanently and/or labelled 'psychotic' because of similar incidents of clinical dehydration. I am sure there are many. Those were extremely hard times for me....I lost my job which we depended on and some very valuable friendships because of my irrational behavior when I was hallucinating and so much more. I will continue as soon as I recover from these sad and quite frankly disturbing memories...

CHAPTER 14

FOCUSED OR NAÏVE?

"The successful warrior is the average man, with laser-like focus."

BRUCE LEE

I am back. I just drank two huge glasses of water which always helps a lot. Now, we will talk about my favorite subject, 'The Brain'. We all know that brain health, mental toughness, great memory, the ability to focus and the ability to make good decisions are most important for survival and for direction in life. Many understand that these things are important. The advisors below all agree that we need these things, however, none will tell us *how* to achieve this mental clarity and focused brain activity.

"Concentration and mental toughness are the margins of victory."

BILL RUSS

The Purple Wave

> *"It takes energy, mental toughness and spiritual reinforcement to successfully deal with life's opportunities and to reach your objectives."*
>
> **ZIG ZIGLAR**

Yes, the brain should or must function well above everything else, after all, it controls the whole body. There is no normal life, without mental fitness. Laird Hamilton has a more direct approach, which I love:

> *"Make sure your worst enemy doesn't live between your own two ears."*
>
> **LAIRD HAMILTON**

These experts know what they are talking about but they can't teach you how to do it, not because they are ignorant or negative people, but they just don't have 'the ultimate tool' to do so. They don't know about Kangen Water®.

We can teach you how to do it. More than that, we can show you how to do it. Besides myself, here are some who already have done it: Canadian World and Olympic Champion, Elvis Stojko (only 50 percent Hungarian-LOL) says he could not do what he did without Kangen Water®. The whole world saw how he performed in the skating rink. Canadian Natural Body Building Champion, Wade T. Lightheart says, he could not have achieved his high goals in such a short time without Kangen Water®. He showed Canada what he can do. Both these athletes claim that Kangen Water® has helped them to do what they did. They don't get paid for endorsements. I met them both. They are very genuine and amazing human beings. They both are working hard to help others and that talks volumes about their character.

> ***"Don't tell me the moon is shining; show me the glint of light on broken glass."***

ANTON CHEKHOV

Lots of energy is used by the brain. Nine trillion nerve cells in the brain, which are 85 percent water, require twenty percent of blood circulation to be allocated. The brain is unique as it is constantly active including during sleep.

Recently, it has been discovered that the human body generates hydro-electric energy when water goes through the cell membranes. The brain uses two mechanisms for its energy requirements. One from food metabolism and creation of sugar, the other from its water supply and conversion of hydroelectric energy, I learned. The body has a delicate balancing system of these two energy sources. This is why when we are dehydrated, sugar cravings intensify. It happens to me and probably many others all the time. More water I drink, less sugar I eat. Of course, the body is much more complicated than this. I just simplified this theory to make it easy to understand, as I think this is a very important point.

To function the way I am and do what I am doing these days, would not have been possible ten years ago. I just did not have the mental sharpness or energy to study and write, travel and learn, read, teach, answer the phone twenty times a day, help countless people and play or skate as I do. To do all that, along with the usual cleaning, cooking, shopping, being a wife, and helping our children? No way! One must be mentally and physically healthy to live this active and wonderful life.

You can do extremely well when you drink water considered to be "the first line of defence for neurological disorders" (Dr. C. Allen), water that "penetrates the blood brain barrier" and water that is energising with no side effects. Did you know that the brain alone uses up at least twenty percent of all the energy of the body? I can testify to that. I should be brutally exhausted while writing this very book for days and nights but I am fine and energised. I am 'enjoying the ride' as I have my water beside me. That's not a joke and neither is it an exaggeration!

Drink water that makes it possible to think better and live better! A fantastic and simple idea!

This is what happened to my dear friend, Roger, who suffered chemical trauma, which ended in PTSD. By switching to Kangen Water® which penetrated his blood brain barrier the brain could heal from the trauma he suffered. I am sure Roger, for nineteen years, 'told' himself to be strong (otherwise he would not have survived) but he couldn't function or work, he couldn't tolerate light, sounds, being around people and he certainly couldn't live and travel the way he does today. He is doing presentations now in front of big crowds and he trains in the gym like a professional athlete. **He got his life back after staying nineteen years in his dark basement.** As fast as in three weeks, drinking Kangen Water® from his cherished SD-501, he started to feel better. He is approachable and shares his amazing story and miraculous recovery with all who are listening. We, Kangen Water® proponents, have nothing to hide, none of us. "We are the product of the product", as Roger says.

Experts are saying that it is not enough to filter tap water. Water having memory, it will remember everything; the additives, the chlorine, the drugs, the fluoride, the entire human history. I know this is quite a lot to take in but it's true.

Water has 'consciousness', which can be difficult to understand or imagine. Water's consciousness was discovered and clearly documented 100 years ago by Victor Schamberger. It is fascinating to consider that the reason your brain is 91 percent water in total is because water is the ultimate receiver and carrier of information. One drop of water can store terabytes of information. The watery content of the brain makes it a far more powerful information processor than any computer. Knowing this, do you really want to have a dried-out brain? Are you complaining that you have bad memory? Who are you blaming for most of your problems? Are you missing out on the different aspects of life because you can't focus? How can a dehydrated brain even remember anything? This is well beyond my understanding.

> *"The story tells that water has a consciousness*
> *that it carries in its memory everything that's*
> *ever happened in this world, from the time*
> *before humans until this moment, which draws*
> *itself in its memory, even as it passes."*
>
> **EMMI ITARANTA**

Quite fascinating are the revelations about water being the medium of consciousness. Evidence suggests that the geometric clustering of water molecules is altered by the subtlest of influences. Bernd Mueller, Director of the Institute of Global Ecology in Portugal, thinks that water even has gender. He states: "When humanity learns how to 'move water' the right way, we will have a different world, a better society". Nature, you see, mirrors society. We find everything we know about in nature: love, trust, partnership, healing and peace.

If we don't maintain and preserve soil integrity, we can't preserve the quality of water, we will only keep destroying it. "Masculine water, which is the rain water, will not be received by the feminine springs of water. This is why water at times turns into violent floods and natural disasters", according to Mr. Mueller. Exciting ideas, which we won't go into in this book, of course.

Let's just agree on the fact that we need to have a well hydrated brain. Our brain cells need to be able to communicate with each other and the rest of the body. That small 'something', that lack of communication in your brain, can put you in a wheelchair. Are you getting it? How many people are in wheelchairs? Only older people used to need them, now more and more kids are stuck in a chair, a permanent cast or something similar as they can't support their own body. Talk to them about water! I do. I want to give them hope.

"We rise by lifting others."

ROBERT INGERSOLL

When a new Kangen water® machine is delivered to a new neighborhood in different cities and people start sharing water, another 'Blue Zone' is forming. How marvellous is that?

The following is just one of the many scientific discoveries that will get you to stop everything you are doing. It will make you turn the TV, PC, FB or your gossiping neighbour off and run to someone who needs this information. This is about the horrible condition labelled as Parkinson's disease. This is what 'updated' medical sites are saying about Parkinson's: *"Although it still isn't clear what exactly causes 'neurodegeneration' in Parkinson's disease, when a significant number of these neurons have died,*

The Purple Wave

the individual will likely start to experience movement-related problems like tremors, rigidity, slowness of movement, and postural instability. These are all hallmark symptoms of Parkinson's disease." No root causes mentioned at all. Why do these neurons die?

Well, here it is; I purposefully copied, 'mot a mot' the text from the published abstract on Pubmed.gov, so you can spread hope, for those with Parkinson's.

"Melanin, a hybrid electronic ionic conductor, may have the potential to split the water molecule into molecular hydrogen and molecular oxygen. Molecular hydrogen is an antioxidant and may be instrumental in preventing the excessive oxidation leading to Parkinson's disease. Melanin, located in the Substantia Nigra, deteriorates in Parkinson's disease so may be related to the development and progression of the disease, since molecular hydrogen would no longer be generated as it deteriorates. Environmental toxins, thought to be related to development of Parkinson's disease, may cause deterioration of intrinsic melanin, since it is a chelator which would collect such environmental contaminants, but its function of splitting the water molecule into molecular hydrogen and oxygen could be affected as a consequence. Restoring melanin function or providing supplemental molecular hydrogen might be potential treatments for Parkinson's disease."

Wow, you might have to read this a few times, it took me a while to get it. I read it six times and I realized that this is huge. Dr. Batmanghelidj calls these neurons "one-time assets". We will come back to this. Are you taking care of your neurons?

Do you know how? Everything I found until now tells me that it is not that difficult. You just have to hydrate your brain and keep the synthetic chemicals and metals away from it. Before the chemical invasion, the pills and tainted foods and such, Alzheimer's was unknown!

You might rightfully ask; What is the connection between Kangen Water® and Molecular Hydrogen?

Yes, I have great news for you. Kangen Water® is loaded with white 'bubbles', which is exactly that; Hydrogen gas.

Molecular Hydrogen is considered the future of medicine by the many experts in the field.

This tiny molecule can penetrate anywhere and everywhere in the body. We will talk about it in more detail but for now, let's enjoy

99

victory! Wow, this is fantastic news. No wonder the list of doctors who are supportive of permanent use of Kangen Water® is growing fast. Now we have tens of thousands of doctors who are embracing our water, not only in Japan but all around the world.

One is Dr. Tim McKnight, M.D. who studied at the Ohio State University College of Medicine. Get this, as it is rare. He also has a PhD in Nutritional Science. He resides in New Philadelphia, Ohio. He states in his book called *"Confessions of a Skeptical Physician "*: *"What I originally dismissed as snake oil hype has developed into a healthy respect and deep interest in the complex nature of water."* Now, he is teaching other doctors and patients about Kangen Water® and its benefits. He was invited, along with a few others, to the White House in May of 2012 to share his knowledge. Another big supporter is Dr. D. Lesman. Again he learned from personal experience. He is a Chiropractor with thirty years of experience from Southern California. He states: *"I'd tried everything and as a last resort I was going to get this for my parents. I started offering them water and it gave them what I couldn't as a physician .... their life back."*

According to quantum theory - get this - the difference between life and death is not so much in the chemistry of the body as it is in organization and structure. Chiropractors who stick with the natural understand this very well.

This is enormous information when you consider that the structure of the water in your body is correlated with sickness, aging and even death. The molecular geometry of the structured water in your body is similar to the structure of crystals like crystalline quartz but in liquid form. Crystalline materials are used in the computer industry because they vibrate at a very precise frequency and so carry signals with amazing speed and precision. I am certain that I vibrate with better precision, LOL, since I am hydrated with superior quality water!

I like the signaling in my brain or what the neurotransmitters are doing. I really do. My thinking is as sharp as a blade, my memory is much better and I can focus better than ever before.

"People often say that motivation doesn't last; well, neither does bathing. That's why we recommend it daily."

ZIG ZIGLAR

Now, you know why we have to drink enough water *daily*. What we are saying is this: we can't store excess water in our body like camels do. Now I just have to prove it to you that 'lack of motivation' is also caused mostly by dehydration. Who knows, it might just be. I know that I am more motivated when I drink enough water. It is all coming from having more energy.

Dr. Corinne Allen (mentioned earlier) has been an international researcher and medical practitioner for over thirty-three years. She is an expert leader in brain disorders in the United States. Dr. Allen has a PhD in nutritional science and lives in California. Using Kangen Water® for over twelve years in her practice, she is having great results treating different personality and mental disorders, behavioural issues, brain traumas, etc. You can listen to her lectures on YouTube but I recommend a fantastic tool, a DVD, which should be in every house in every country, no matter who you are. It is called: "The Science & Practical Uses of ERW in Brain and Neurological Issues."

How clever to use Kangen Water® as a tool when it comes to the brain!

I met Dr. Allen in Vegas in 2018 and I remember her saying how many people are not aware about the behavioural problems and mental issues that are almost always a result of inflammation in the brain after accidents or trauma. Physical, chemical or emotional trauma is very hard on the brain and until now, these problems could not be helped as no medication could even touch the broken areas of the brain without doing further damage. *"But hydrogen molecules, being so tiny, can actually penetrate the blood brain barrier,"* she says. Because of the anti-inflammatory and anti-oxidant properties of the hydrogen in the water, the affected area of the brain can heal.

Often (not in every case, but often) with the 'water treatment', people's mental issues just disappear and their behavior normalizes again. Marvellous. I think this is huge and beautiful. We all know how big the 'PTSD' issue is. Thousands commit suicide because they can't get better from Post Traumatic Stress Disorder (inflammation caused in the brain by the trauma) and often because of the concoction of prescription drugs they are put on regularly. These mess with the brain and often cause greater issues.

Dr. Allen is also having great results with autistic children.

Parents need to know about this! Sodas and lack of water are destroying these children.

She states: *"Children with autism often are dangerously dehydrated and neglected, their brain function compromised, as they don't drink water."*

"People who need help sometimes look a lot like people who don't need help."

GLENNON MELTON

Now we have a new tool to change people's lives and make it better, much better. Many people could be helped if this was common knowledge. Dr. Allen achieved as much as forty-three percent improvement (this is unheard of) with children who have different forms of autism. She also treats Asperger's, ADD, Dyslexia, learning disabilities, PTSD and all stress-related illnesses at her clinic called, "SHILOH Institute, Center for Brain and Body Wellness". She saves lots a money for people with brain issues. Why spend thousands on a dead-end diagnosis with no solutions?

This next story validated what I've learned from Dr. Corinne Allen.

M. was a teenager who was hit by a truck while riding his bicycle. The traumas from this accident really affected him and, of course, his behaviour. Everything went wrong with him. He could not study any longer, he was hard to handle and he started drinking, smoking and doing light drugs after he was put on medication. He refused the meds many times as he was tormented by the horrible side effects. He did not work, did not go to school or live according to his family's norm. He did not have much of a future. When I heard about this tragic situation, I invited his mom to see our presentation. She was a client of mine at the time. We became friends after this incident. Thankfully she came and listened. She immediately realised that her son could be helped by this medical device. She purchased the machine and started her son on the water. We also replaced the pills with UKON, our turmeric superfood. He became easier to get along with, very soon after. We all embraced him and my husband was mentoring and supervising him for a month. We spent some time with him. He was constantly improving mentally. He started working soon after this. He slowly reduced his alcohol consumption to social drinking. Now, four years later, he is twenty-two and he is a hard-working young man who is most definitely looking at a great future. He has clear goals now, listens to motivational videos, interacts with people and chooses friends wisely. He is on his way to quit smoking completely. This precious young man thankfully has become a pillar in the family. When I see M., I always remember how much our water is needed as it really does work.

> *"What mental health needs is more sunlight, more candor, more unashamed conversation."*
>
> **GLENN CLOSE**

Think about the quality of the water, which will increase not only the energy to your brain, but also the clarity or the quality of your thoughts... "We might go so far as to say that you should not only think about Kangen Water®, but that **you could be thinking with Kangen Water®,** says Dr. Mona Harrison, MD. Dr. Harrison received her medical training at the University of Maryland, Harvard University and the Boston University Medical Centers. She specialises in pediatrics, previously holding the title of Chief Medical Officer at Washington DC General Hospital. She states: *"Cysts are the beginning of tumors, which lead to cancer because minerals are deficient from that part of the body. Cancer is a long period of mineral deficiency caused by an over-acidic condition of the body."* This is precisely why we and all our friends who own a machine almost never drink any of the other drinks out there, except Kangen Water®. They are all acidic and will contribute to the acidity of the body more than anything else. We have this vital information. Sadly, most of the people don't. Only we can change that. No wonder, so many people are having cognitive issues these days, problems with coordination, concentration and nerve transmission. All these are serious, often debilitating conditions.

I would add to this my own personal experience. It is much easier to think 'positive' when your brain is functioning at its best capacity.

> *"It is well for the heart to be naïve, and for the mind not to be."*
>
> **ANATOLE FRANCE**

CHAPTER 15

A MODERN-DAY NIGHTMARE

"I don't paint dreams or nightmares.
I paint my own reality."

FRIDA KAHLO

The worst 'nightmare' I have ever experienced happened (unfortunately it really happened) in my thirties when I became the 'victim' of a well-meaning dentist. I never liked the term, I always refused to be a victim. This time, in my desperate attempt to stay alive, I ended up visiting twenty-eight doctors and healers in a period of eight years. I have not only medical records, but Court records, as well to prove it. I experienced firsthand how deficient the system is. Then I came to a huge realisation and that realisation, which I call 'the light', saved my life.

The inconvenient truth I realised was that my health is not a doctor's issue, it is my own responsibility.

The Purple Wave

*"Real transformation requires real honesty!
If you want to move forward,
get real with yourself."*

BRYANT MCGILL

After 'waking up', I immediately took responsibility. No one had to convince me to take 'the road less travelled'. I understood the logic. It was simple common sense. I had to look inwards to figure out what happened to me in the last five years that could have had this horrible effect on my health. Me not being well, affected my son's health, also. My attention switched from my kids towards myself. Not a great thing for a mother.

If you are a wife or a mother, you are responsible for everyone's health as *the main nourisher* of the family. I also realised this truth. I had to be a mother before anything else.

My son wasn't doing well academically so I started to look into my son's eating habits. I made sure he was not getting any junk and eating healthy meals every day. My son's 'behaviour', his mental attitude and academic capacity turned 180 degrees when I cleaned his room out of junk (bags and bags of candy and chips, pizza boxes and such) and he started to supplement with the best vitamins. Fresh fruits and veggies were mandatory to eat again, every day and every night as a snack. There was a huge change in his energy level in less than three months. It turned out that he wasn't 'lazy' after all, he just had no energy being so tall and not having adequate nutrients in his diet. It makes me sad because I know that many people today will never be healthy or successful in life (meaning happy and capable of providing for their families) simply because of lack of water and nutrition. Please read the book called: "Is your child's brain starving?" by Dr. Michael R. Lyon, MD.

A Naturopath doctor in Abbotsford, Dr. Ewing, saved my life. He discovered the massive loads of mercury and a few other toxic metals in my system through special testing. This was caused mostly by the eight amalgam fillings and numerous root canals in my mouth as well as some second-hand smoke I'd endured for three years while working in an office of smokers in Romania.

Thirty years have passed since I was so ill and the system did not learn anything. Over thirty years passed since my mom developed cirrhosis and cancer of the liver from prescription drugs and the system learned nothing. Thankfully, I did but the naïve patient today still goes in with symptoms of toxicity from poisons, insufficient water and nutrients, lack of Vitamin D and other ailments that potentially could be cured by proper care but they just get prescribed more poison!

It is a well-known fact that mercury and many other heavy metals are toxic and cause serious health issues. The symptoms caused by these metals, things like chest pain and panic attacks, cramps and spasms, are real and scary. Heavy metal poisoning requires special testing and this is not acknowledged or covered by mainstream medical care.

Isn't it revolting that the very system, which should help us to stay healthy is causing more and often bigger problems?

I stay away from everything unnatural, like pills, tanning salons, flu shots, and most vaccines, etc. My family physician - yes, I have one - is an extraordinary doctor. He is not the typical pill pusher. I am very blessed. He has a message in his computer. It says: "Mrs. Klara Reid doesn't accept prescription drugs!" - end of message. This makes things less complicated between me and the possible 'replacement' doctors if he is away.

Eighty percent of heart attacks in people under forty are caused by oxidation, the root cause being heavy metals, stress, and dehydration. This is according to official autopsy results shared with me by my bio-dentist who removed all the amalgam from my mouth. The top six sources of heavy metals and toxic aluminium are: amalgam, prescription drugs, vaccines, chlorine, pesticides and baking powder. Just so you know. Dehydration makes toxicity with these compounds detrimental. This is what nearly killed me.

Thankfully, specialists who can take care of these issues exist outside of the system. Talk to a good nutritionist who has the knowledge to guide you through healing with real food, not synthetic pills. I found one. She is young, but her very grateful clientele is growing fast. I will reveal her name a bit later.

If you don't understand how your body works, how are you going to take care of it?

Who will you believe? The person who tells you that you need Lipitor or the person who says that Lipitor is causing more heart attacks than Cholesterol? The TV-Ad, which tells you to take Lipitor or the TV-Ad of

The Purple Wave

the local Lawyer who tells you that you have a case in the event you are 'injured' from Lipitor?

"Confusion is a word we have invented for an order which is not yet understood."

UNKNOWN

This is why you need to know yourself what is going on. I know who to believe. Do you see it now? Read the book called "The Cholesterol Conspiracy" by Dr. Ladd McNamara. He graduated from the University of Texas Medical school in Dallas, in 1989. From 1993 he practiced medicine in Atlanta, specialising in Gynecology, Laparoscopy, Menopausal Management and Anti-Aging medicine. Dr. McNamara has been published in Medical Journals, Medical books and Manuscripts on the topic of Anti-Ageing and Nutraceutical Medicine. He retired from mainstream medicine (disgusted from it, I am sure!) in 2003.

According to many doctors and experts, the body 'makes' cholesterol to protect itself from oxidation. That I believe and you will too as we will investigate and the ultimate proof will be shared here soon. We have an amazing body. So, oxidation is the root cause of 'bad' cholesterol, which is not the same for everyone, so no one can tell what is the normal amount for you. We see many cases when people get killed faster and more often from cholesterol lowering drugs than cholesterol itself.

The medical system is so ineffective, in fact, that a whole new industry has developed. We have holistic practitioners who try to undo the harmful things dentists and doctors did (or in many cases, didn't do; they just got paid for it...). Getting things 'undone' cost me over $50,000. What if someone doesn't have that kind of money or the proper information? Yes, they just suffer and die.

Because of this, the whole economy is affected. Our governments are going to collapse due to our faulty medical system.

Do you understand where the landmines are hidden? If not, please learn fast! Otherwise, I assure you, they will blow up right in your face and you won't even know what hit you! I see this every day. I learned what I know from experience and from rare books that, sadly, are not on library shelves. Libraries are more controlled than you might think!

We should communicate more openly so we can get to the bottom of things. How would you like to be able to 'neutralise' all your life's stresses before they destroy your health? Do you know how to shop for food and perhaps take the smart phone away from the three-year-old? You would be smarter than the 'smartphone' if you did.

> ### *"The only fence against the world is a thorough knowledge of it."*
>
> **JOHN LOCKE**

One of the biggest mistakes we make is when we underestimate the power we have as consumers. Whatever is sold is bought. People are buying into everything that is sold. What a nonsense! The truth is whatever is bought is sold. If we don't buy it, how they can sell it? I understand that it is hard to believe that things are this simple. Everyone wants to convince us that health and wellbeing are complicated, and that you need them or their products.

But much of what is sold is harmful or it doesn't work. I consider, for example, all that is called 'Sunblock' another modern-day nightmare. First, they sell you sunblock, which poisons the fish of the sea and then they sell you vitamin D, which you should be getting from sunshine! Does this make sense to you? Can you imagine something so powerful that it stops the Sun and it won't hurt you? I can't. The fish die from it, yet people are puzzled where cancer is coming from? People spray their kids with that poison at the beach. Outrageous! When poor kids finally are about to get some vitamin D from the sun, the parents stop this so needed natural process. Those parents aren't normal in my eyes. Sorry, but I have to be honest. There is an intelligent way to get sun gradually and not to get burned! How about putting your kids to bed at 8:00 p.m. and get them out to the beach at 8:00 am until, let's say 11:00 a.m.? Oh, but that would ruin the movie night, which kept them up late the night before. So, they arrive at the beach at noon and they spend money on toxic chemicals! They are not allergic to the sun! They are 'protected' from the sun most of the year. Lack of natural sunlight, sun, lack of water and lack of discipline are the causes why they can't handle the sun, which they badly need!

Natural vitamin D is not fully replaceable!

Being over-sensitive to the sun is a sure indication of big-time dehydration!

"But once in a while, you pick the right thing, the exact best thing. Every day the moment you open your eyes and pull off your blankets, that's what you hope for: The sunshine on your face, warm enough to make your heart sing."

SARAH OCKLER

Let the children's hearts sing by getting lots a sunshine! Drop the nasty sunblock forever. I have been a true worshipper of the Sun ever since I was a child. I always made time for being in the Sun. I know that the Sun healed me many times. I would not be here today if not for the Sun. From three months up, my kids had sunbathing included in their daily routine. I made sure that they get two hours or so of the morning or the afternoon Sun, daily. People today don't have time to be outdoors when the Sun is shining. Major landmine just like the lack of natural salt is**.**

Salt accumulates in your body only when it is not flushed out due to lack of water!

Salt completely dissolves in water. Drinking enough water will eliminate the excess salt. You should eat salt freely, as much as your body requires. Instead of adding water to your diet, most doctors advise you to drop the salt. Another horrible 'medical advice'! I recommend a You Tube video called; *"Water, Natural Salt and Exercise, in that order"* by Dr. Batmanghelidj. It was an eye opener for me. Please don't confuse natural, whole spectrum salt containing all the 80 plus minerals, with sodium, which is used in canned foods, etc. That white powder, just like the other white powders (refined sugar, baking soda, white-bleached flour, artificial sweeteners) is dangerous. This product is a 'leftover' from real salt after the precious minerals are taken out in order to sell them separately. Greed, Greed and more greed!

It is a war out there and you won't even notice it if you are preoccupied with your electronic toys and other distractions.

Most people are not comfortable talking about their health until the day comes when they are told: "You need to start chemo right away, or you will die in six months!" Even then they won't wake up. This is called the "Nocebo effect". In medicine, a Nocebo is something that creates harmful effects in a patient. Conversely, a Placebo is an inert substance or form of therapy that creates a beneficial response in a person. Cancer doctors give you a nocebo to scare you into treatments and like a fish, you take the bait! (chemo, surgery or radiation—all they know). How sad. Instead of the 'six months prognosis' according to author and motivational speaker, Les Brown, oncologists should tell their patients that *"Their knowledge and capability are terminated, so they can't help the patient any longer."* I agree. To say anything else to a person with a 'terminal illness' is reckless, ridiculous and unethical. Les Brown was speaking on stage fifteen years after a doctor told him that he had two years maximum to live. No comment! This 'terminal illness' BS, which by the way, doesn't exist (except in very rare cases) is sold through movies a lot, lately. (Why shouldn't they? Hollywood is doing everything else immoral!) People are programmed and they die exactly when they are told that they should die! They have no idea that cancer can be reversed. I will never forget Dr. Day, this amazing woman, whose breast cancer was so advanced that they thought that she would die that night. Dr. Lorraine Day reversed her severe, advanced cancer by rebuilding her immune system by natural therapies, so her body could heal itself. The key was that she did not accept any medication or poisonous treatment, she trusted her body and only ate alkalising, organic, raw vegetables.

*"It is courage, courage, courage, that raises
the blood of life to crimson splendor..."*

HORACE

The Purple Wave

Dr. Day is an internationally acclaimed orthopedic trauma surgeon and author of a few absolutely fabulous books who was associated with the University of California, San Francisco, School of Medicine for fifteen years. She was also Chief of Orthopedic Surgery at San Francisco General Hospital. She has been invited to lecture extensively throughout the U.S. and the world and has appeared on numerous radio and television shows including 60 minutes, Nightline, Larry King Live, The 700 Club, etc. Dr. Day is my hero. Her courage gives hope for millions. I had the privilege to listen to her lecture at a Health Show.

Please read the book: *"Killing Cancer, Not People"* by Robert Wright to get the information you need for prevention and truly effective natural treatments for cancer. This book is vital in case you want to avoid becoming the next victim of the cancer industry! Anyone can order the book from the website. You will also receive an amazing free newsletter from Bob with updated information about health in general. This includes of course most of the degenerative and immune problems as well. I wish that I'd had this information years ago when my mom was ill. If I could only recommend one eye-opening book, this would be it!

"There are many who don't wish to sleep for fear of nightmares. Sadly, there are many who don't wish to wake for the same reason."

RICHELLE GOODRICH

We've all got two choices. We can either bury our head in the sand or we can open our eyes and minds and see.

CHAPTER 16

LESSONS FROM HISTORY

"We spend a great deal of time studying history which, let's face it, is mostly the history of stupidity."

STEPHEN HAWKING

My naivety - what was left of it - was terminated in about two days when I first read Bob's book and got involved with the *American Anti-Cancer Institute*. Robert Wright or "Bob" (how he calls himself) is straight forward, he's bold and he's right on the money. People with integrity like Bob who can impart wisdom and uncompromised information are rare and priceless. He walks the walk and he shares his valuable knowledge, the work of a lifetime, free of charge.

Now, I would like to go back in time and look at some important lessons we can learn from history. The smart thing to do is to learn from others, not by going through the ordeal ourselves.

I will mention only two of the many lessons we should never forget!

In 1850, a caring obstetrician, a practically unknown physician who wasn't part of the establishment (and to make it worse, a Hungarian Jew) named Ignaz Semmelweis (yes, another Hungarian—Sorry, I assure

The Purple Wave

you I am not doing it on purpose) stepped on the podium of the medical society in Vienna and shouted: "Wash your hands!" He had a revelation about what was causing the devastating epidemic called 'child bed fever'. He cared deeply about the mothers who were dying, leaving hundreds of orphans behind and this agony helped him to find the root cause of one of history's greatest tragedies. Hundreds of mothers were dying soon after they gave birth. He started advising his colleagues to wash and disinfect their hands.

Did anyone listen? The medical establishment not only ignored everything he was saying, but ridiculed him, driving him insane until he ended up in a mental institution. Wouldn't you if you knew exactly how to save multiple lives, millions of lives and no one would listen? What was happening was the doctors who worked on dead bodies doing autopsies in the mornings, kept delivering babies in the afternoons and with their dirty hands, they infected the mothers causing sepsis.

It was no epidemic. It was a simple problem. The elite of the doctors were both the cause and potential solution. But they thought the solution was too simple and so they didn't listen**.**

I call this the hazard of the complicated mind.

Again, this went on for decades and many more women died creating a whole pool of babies without moms to care for them. Can you think about a more tragic story than this? Sadly, history is repeating itself. Today, the majority is not suspecting, nor believing that a simple thing like cellular dehydration and an overly toxic body can be the cause of chronic illnesses and such a staggering number of premature deaths.

*"History repeats itself, because no one
was listening the first time."*

ANONYMOUS

Another example is scurvy. Around 1520, many sailing ships on Europe's trade routes began losing hundreds of sailors to what people believed to be an 'epidemic'. The symptoms of the disease where so horrible that doctors believed these men were dying of syphilis, cholera, or something similar. Years later, it was discovered that simply deficiency of vitamins killed them because the sailors did not eat anything fresh for months. Just eating limes or lemons (Vitamin C) could have saved their lives. Today, we know that Vitamin B and/or C deficiency is extremely harmful but for all those sailors who died, the life saving revelation came too late. Are you getting it? We have a somewhat similar situation with water dinking today, I think. Those who are ill today or dying have to be helped now! If you are dehydrated now, you need this information NOW!

The time for medical grade water is here and those who know this have a moral obligation to tell others about it.

(This is why at age 60, I switched careers. Who does such a thing? Only a crazy woman like Klara.) I really believe that morals should come before money.

"The value of history, is indeed, not scientific, but moral, by liberalizing the mind, by deepening the sympathies, by fortifying the will, it enables us to control, not society, but ourselves - a much more important thing..."

CARL BECKER

We should avoid the mistakes of the past but are we up to the challenge?

Well-known brain surgeon, Dr. Ben Carson says "The populous doesn't understand the basics of their health and because of it they are easily manipulated." Dr. Carson is retired from Medicine, lives in the United States and became a public servant after being a presidential candidate in 2016.

There are thousands of doctors who are saying that the population is chronically dehydrated, toxic and acidic. This leads to a compromised immune system. There is no cancer or autoimmune disorder epidemic, yet millions die because of this great confusion.

It dos not matter, if its cancer, a super-bug, an engineered bio-weapon, a virus, more EMF pollution or stress, there are natural solutions to regain your health, some simpler and more efficient than others. Another wonderful book caught my attention. It is called: "After the Doctors... What Can You Do?" I would call it: Before the Doctors... What Should You Do! If people knew how to look after their bodies, oh, that would make life so much better and easier. 500 years after scurvy [2020 V 1520] history repeats itself one again. Vitamins and minerals, like vitamin D, C, B, K, A and Zinc are more effective than masks, ventilators, social distancing or other crazy initiatives. This information is coming from honest and serious doctors, not from corrupt politicians. I meet so many people who are after cancer protocols like chemo and such. They are saying that if they knew then what they know now, they would do everything differently.

You know your own body best. Detoxing is most definitely not fun; however, it is the only lasting way of getting your health back. It worked for me and many others I know! There are many ways to detox and get rid of the different poisons. Drinking Kangen Water® is the fastest and easiest way to do that. For certain things like heavy metals you will need more than water. Natural chlorophyll is one of those amazing remedies. Then, you need to rebuild your immune system naturally with wholesome nutrients and a change in lifestyle so it won't happen again! Change your habits! Get out of a poisonous relationship, do whatever you have to do. Until you wake up and see this simple reality, you cannot be helped.

This is a practical and cost-effective way to get rid of the accumulated poisons in the body, restoring this way the body's sensitive pH balance. It will also hydrate you like nothing else on Earth. We are 75 percent water so taking care of the cell water and our digestive system will help the body to get at least 75 percent better.

That is much more than any other remedy, natural or synthetic can do.

Real science is advancing all the time. These revelations come on a regular basis. The problem is that it can be challenging to find them.

Scientists have discovered that the water environment of both cancerous and diabetic cells is less structured. Accordingly, both cancer and diabetes have a common feature; the destruction of water structure at the cellular level. I think this discovery is phenomenal. There are doctors and scientists today who really understand how the body works. They are loud! *"You are not sick, you are thirsty!"* says Dr. Batmanghelidj while Dr. Baroody is also shouting *"Alkalize or die!"* Sherry A. Rogers *tells you straight! "Detoxify or die!"* These titles should wake up everyone. I love Dr. Gabor Lenkei, a medical doctor in Hungary (Oops-not again! *Not another Hungarian!?)* Anyway, Dr. Lenkei is actually traveling from city to city and from village to village telling people that what they need is water, not prescription drugs. One of his many books is called *"Cenzurazott Egeszseg".* No worries! I am translating it to you right away. Here it is;

"*Censored Health*". This book is original, hilarious and simply amazing. The medical authorities are after him now harassing the good doctor to silence him. What a world we live in!

Thank God there are quite a few doctors out there who are not part of the 'system' who are knowledgeable and willing. One of them is Dr. Zoltan Rona who is practicing Complementary or as he calls it Integrative Medicine in Canada, and is an expert in nutritional biochemistry. We are blessed by him and his colleagues and the information they share. It might be risky for them to speak up, they need our support and prayers, along with Bob Wright. The number of doctors who have the courage to speak up is frighteningly small.

Wade Lightheart's book (pure Canadian not Hungarian!) *"Staying Alive in a Toxic World"* is a great book and what a great title. Friends, everyone needs constant detoxification "to stay alive" in today's environment. Are you plugged in? Health won't be delivered to you. A Kangen® Machine, however, will be delivered in two days by UPS! You just have to ask. We must look after ourselves if we want to live, I learned. This is one of the reasons why I consider ERW the most significant tool for great health. It is helping me manage my delicate health. This is the best option I ever had for the permanent heart damage and a bunch of already forgotten auto-immune disorders I have had to deal with. Once you get as ill as I did, you will always have a compromised immune system so you really have to watch what you are doing! I am so grateful for this water.

"Divine health begins with Gratitude."

DR. PARTHA NANDI

I know a few people who travel every three years and pay something like $20,000 and more to 'detox' at special clinics, often outside of Canada or the USA. Others pay $250,000 for a new liver so they can live. For some, paying a ridiculously low amount for the best source of water, which will detox and hydrate the entire family for twenty five or so years is 'too expensive.'

The same device, which is producing drinking water, can also be used to make food cleaner, safer, tastier and help the environment by

The Purple Wave

eliminating plastics and chemicals. It really puzzles me when people don't get it. Which part sounds tricky to you? Some, I think are just very 'different' in their thinking. I hope I am not offending anyone!

Slowly but surely (I hope you noticed) I am introducing to you the exact 'tool', which we all so desperately need. A surprise, which should not surprise you. Solutions like this happen once in 200 years when common sense goes wild. Why? **Because we are limited in our thinking most of the time but at times we act with our hearts and souls, we create out of compassion and then we get it right.**

I know that the Kangen® machine was born out of compassion. I can feel it. Love transcends. We share the water for the same reason because of compassion. I think the rejection we see at times is solely because of Ego. Our ego, at times, tells us that we know better and we already know everything. Nothing can be further from the truth. When I thought that I knew everything about natural approaches, Kangen Water® taught me a huge lesson.

How was this idea born? I was puzzled. Was it looking back to imitate nature's water or looking ahead predicting upcoming problems with the source water? Perhaps all of the above. Kangen® in Japanese indeed means: "Back to Origin".

Where do you find this water, how do you find it when thousands of different kinds are advertised? How did I find it? I didn't. How could I? I wasn't looking. The water found me. I can only thank GOD for it. Now it has found you. The beautiful part is that we don't have to rely on a store, a person or anyone! We can produce it. This is probably the most fantastic information I can ever share with you. Now you know that a very simple change in your lifestyle like changing your water and adjusting your water intake will have a profound impact on your overall health.

Are you asking the question "How can I produce it?"

Well, today, we solve most of our problems with computers or technology, don't we? One small personal computer will do many of the jobs of the past. Wouldn't it be amazing if we could come up with a 'computer', if you will, to take care of our health! Some are thinking: *Oh, that will never happen! That is just impossible!* Are you losing hope? Please don't.

*"There was never a night or a problem
that could defeat sunrise or hope."*

BERNARD WILLIAM

CHAPTER 17

WHAT? A HEALTH MACHINE?

*"Every once in a while, a new technology,
an old problem and a big idea turn
into an innovation."*

DEAN CAMEN

Yes, this is probably what happened. An old problem, a new technology and a big idea mysteriously met. So, now I can tell you that a computerised system already exists, the ultimate health machine has already been invented and it is available to anyone who is interested.

The Kangen® machine is not an idea any longer. The "big idea" turned into an innovation. It came to life and it is working. This technological marvel, this triumph of human ingenuity is producing water at my home as we speak, all day long. This water will alkalize you, hydrate you, detox you and reduce oxidation in your cells so it takes care of most problems that life throws at you. That includes stress.

We don't have to carry 'holy water' from kilometers away, we just have to drink it. We don't have to spend money every day, we just have to

The Purple Wave

drink it. We don't have to worry about our family members, we just have to ask them to drink it. How you ask? You show it to them by drinking the water yourself. They will notice the difference in you!

This water completely changed our lives. This water gives us tons of energy daily. I have a tendency toward 'road rage' so driving the car on highways always caused extreme stress for me. I make sure that I have my water with me and I drink. Before the free radicals start the chain reaction and cause damage in my body, I have already neutralised the harmful effects of this crazy stress. No acidity, no inflammation! No inflammation, no pain!

> *"Technology, like art, is a soaring*
> *exercise of the human imagination."*
>
> **DANIEL BELL**

The cyst I had under my arm for thirty years (ever since I was breastfeeding my babies) disappeared in only three weeks. The chronic fatigue I was dealing with for decades, completely went away. Besides the tremendous energy, the water had an alkalizing effect on me. I think this is huge! We know how hard it is to be on a vegan, organic raw diet to achieve an alkaline body. The acidity of my urine changed almost instantly and the acid reflux disappeared. No more urinary tract infections or bladder infections for seven years now. Those were happening almost monthly. No more asthma puffers for me, 95 percent of allergies are gone and no trouble sleeping. (I was told that I had sleep apnea, which I intentionally ignored.) During the second year of faithfully drinking the water, soon after I saw what this water can do I got involved and started to immerse myself in the study of it.

Kangen Water® has a beautiful colour because of the high pH of the water. You can see this if you put pH drops into it. So, how do pH drops work? A pH drop is "a halochromic chemical compound" added in small amounts to a solution so the acidity or basicity of the solution can be determined visually. The 'pH indicator' in fact is a 'chemical detector' of positively charged hydrogen ions (H+).

We named this water, which made us feel so great so fast, "The Purple Wave" because the 9.5 water has a vivid, purple colour, - the exact colour that 9.5 pH alkalinity should show on the pH chart. When we add Kangen Water® to a glass of bottled or tap water, that acidic liquid will turn from yellow into purple. This shows how potent this water is and how easily it will change the pH of our body fluids, as well. Sodas are so acidic, however, that even Kangen Water® cannot help. They show an orange colour, which is about 2.5 pH. Please note that chemically-made 'alkaline' water doesn't have the power to alkalise the body. So, when your doctor tells you that alkaline water is not good for you, he is right! He is referring to chemically altered water (which might interfere with your stomach acid). Kangen Water® or ERW is naturally alkalised. Huge difference! The alkalinity however, is not the most important quality of this water. There is something totally unique and extraordinary here and that is what transformed the purple wave into a 'tsunami'! It's called Molecular Hydrogen, or Hydrogen gas. That's right.

*"Some piously record "In the beginning God",
but I say in the beginning Hydrogen."*

HARLOW SHAPLEY

A few extremely fortunate, slowly but surely found out about Molecular Hydrogen, which is nothing short of a miracle.

We will see what this is in the next chapter. The masses have no idea about this, not yet. You must know about this. This 'tsunami' is not on the news, at least not in this country, so pay attention to the research and scientific facts. While the mainstream media is not mentioning the hydrogen story, the Huffington Post has taken an active interest once. Too little, too late? It is not too late for you, now you know about it. The Huffington Post commented about Molecular Hydrogen in 2016 and they brought the potential ability of hydrogen rich water to reduce free radical activity to the attention of the public, but usually not many are paying attention to such a 'boring' news.

The Purple Wave

In the article, Dr. Lee states: *"The more I learn about Hydrogen the more dedicated and passionate I become in educating and helping others."* So am I, but I don't have the impressive credentials he has:

- 1987-1993 M.B. Medical Science, Wonju College of Medicine, Yonsei University, Wonju, Korea

- 2001-2005 Instructor, Department of Parasitology, Wonju College of Medicine, Yonsei University

- 2005-2008 Assistant Professor, Department of Parasitology, Wonju College of Medicine, Yonsei University

- 2010-present President of The Korean Water Society

- 2013-present Full Professor, Department of Environmental Medical Biology, Wonju College of Medicine, Yonsei University... and much more but we can save trees if we stop now...

Be aware as fake hydrogen water is also flooding the marketplace just as fake alkaline water did. The 'hydrogen machine' looks like a tea kettle, you have to fill it up with water. It is definitely not a medical device. You won't be able to create different pH waters. Just to make hydrogen, I personally would never pay $1,500 or more. When we measured the pH of this water, it had the same pH as the tap water and had no negative charge! How can that be healthy? We are back to square one. It is amazing how fast 'copycats' catch up with trends. Before you realise it, they grabbed your money.

Hydrogen, the lightest element on the periodic table, which is the most abundant substance in the universe, has been completely overlooked, however, this new discovery about Molecular Hydrogen is causing waves for a good reason. Only since 2007 we do know about this, so don't be surprised if you (or your doctor) haven't heard about it, just yet. We will talk more about Hydrogen gas and what it does in the next chapter.

You can drink a gallon of Kangen Water® in one sitting and you won't feel it in your stomach. It is truly magical. This magic has a scientific explanation indeed, which is coming soon. In my opinion, many experts correctly suspect that structured water is the key to DNA signaling, enzyme activity and so on. I am not sure how much we, humans, understand about DNA and enzymes but I am sure that more discoveries will come as water indeed is mysterious. I am also sure that these discoveries will change the face of medicine and the landscape of health care.

"You never change things by fighting the existing reality, to change something, build a new model that will make the existing model obsolete."

BUCKMINSTER FULLER

Kangen Water® is changing the field of medicine not by fighting the existing procedures or treatments but by replacing them!
Only real stuff has that power.
Please look for 'Electrolyzed Reduced Water' or 'Molecular Hydrogen' at (www.googlescholar.com), (www.pubmed.gov), the only places where you will find verified or reliable information when it comes to the Internet.
This is a *'biological'* form of water- considered so because it is consistent with our cell water.
There are over 400 human diseases and disease models and over 1000 peer reviewed scientific abstracts about molecular hydrogen's therapeutic effects that anyone can research if they have the time and the ambition.

I also learned that water can be highly organized (structured) forming a liquid crystalline matrix, which has been found to surround healthy DNA and other healthy proteins in the body or it can be un-organized as is the water that surrounds cancerous cells and abnormal DNA.

There is so much unknown about how this works, yet certain things about water have been well-known for centuries.

'Bulk water' is messed up, has no structure (lost its structure); perhaps this is the biggest reason, I am thinking, why most of us have no desire to drink it!

There is a paradigm shift in science today, as more and more people are becoming interested in these ideas. It is not hard to guess why. Understanding water is an important part of our past, it should be part

The Purple Wave

of our present and it will definitely be part of our future. It is not hard to fall in love with water once we pay attention to it.

> *"Science is not only a disciple of reason,*
> *but also, one of romance and passion."*
>
> **STEPHEN HAWKING**

CHAPTER 18

THE ESSENCE

"Nature is so powerful, so strong. Capturing its essence is not easy - your work becomes a dance with light and the weather. It takes you to a place within yourself."

ANNIE LEIBOVITZ

I will make the attempt. If I can make this boring chapter fun and easy to capture the essence of Kangen Water®, I may deserve a nomination for a Pulitzer prize, or something. LOL.

We all understand the storms, lightning, wind and movement in nature. Inspired by nature, there is a lot going on in the ioniser unit, as well. In order to create this 'storm', a continuous direct current is required as electrolysis doesn't just happen. We have to 'force it'. When this kind of power 'zaps' the water, we can expect substantial structural changes. If this is too much for you, or boring, please proceed to the next chapter.

I would like to remind you that I am not a scientist, I am a story teller and I can only give you as much as I understand, however, I needed to know what was happening in the machine. I wanted to understand why Kangen Water® did what it did for me and my friend Roger.

124

The way I see it, understanding ERW is not easy, but it is not complicated, either. It is one of those things. You either understand it or you just drink the water. Either way, Kangen Water® as a medical grade water is real and it is working for all who are drinking it. Now, let's examine what is really happening during the 'storm' inside the ioniser. Water gains life from nature. The storm that is created in the ionizer will 'revitalise' the water the same way as it happens in nature. The waters 'polluted' memory will also be erased and that is a game changer.

What is unique about water, which turns it into a 'universal solvent' is its tendency to form hydrogen bonds not only within its own molecule, but either with other water molecules or different (other than water) molecules, as well.

A mysterious and crazy dancing and bouncing is going on constantly in the water. Salt or other organics can be dissolved in water because of this unique bonding ability of the hydrogen in the water molecule.

Water is the medium for life sustaining reactions in all living systems but also an active component of these reactions.

The water molecule contains two hydrogen and one oxygen atom as you probably already know. The hydrogen atom only contains one proton, which is positively charged and one electron, which is negatively charged. Oxygen on the other hand contains eight protons in its core called the nucleus and eight (four sets of two, paired) electrons revolving around its nucleus. These atoms unite and form water or 'split' (disassociate) and form ions. The hydrogen atom is capable of ionizing simply by losing its electron and becoming an isolated proton and of course will have a positive charge as all protons are positive (H+).

"Exploration is really the essence
of the human spirit."

FRANK BORMAN

The hydrogen atom while remaining covalently bonded to the oxygen of its own molecule can form a weak bond with the oxygen of another molecule. Because of this we can create electronegative and electropositive charge and the water becomes a continuous chemical entity. This bonding keeps happening constantly.

This *rearrangement* of the weak bonds of the water molecule is in essence the 'chemistry of life'.

In the case of ionization, we are are talking about more of a 'structural' and/or electrical change than a chemical one. During ionization we are witnessing removals or additions of electrons.

- **When the 'removal' of an electron happens, not only electronegative or electropositive charge is created but oxidation as well.**

- **When an 'addition' happens, we call that reduction, during which energy is stored in the reduced compound.**

- **When oxidation happens, energy is liberated. When one substance is oxidised, the other is reduced. This is called "redox" reaction.**

- **The accumulation or higher concentration of hydrogen ions (H+) leads to an acidic substance.**

- **The accumulation or higher concentration of hydroxide ions (OH-) leads to alkalinity in a solution.**

  This acid - alkaline balance is measured in pH (possible Hydrogen). The pH chart goes to fourteen. (1-14) Seven is neutral, less than seven means acidic, more than seven means alkaline.

At seven, the donations in the water are equal.

The pH is extremely important because everything 'living' is sensitive to pH. Mostly all parts of the body function well only if the pH is slightly alkaline. Our blood is so crucial to be slightly alkaline that the body is designed to keep it there between 7.365-7.4 pH. Out of this range coma or death occurs. Most of the body fluids, the lymphatic system, for example, (the extra cellular water) should be around 7.2-7.3 pH. Numerous mechanisms aid the body in stabilising its fluids' pH level. The substances called 'buffers', also help to stabilize the pH. These buffers have the capacity to bond or release ions, depending on the need. Biochemical reactions either release or use up ions.

The Purple Wave

The properties of the water from the pH standpoint is important but not nearly as important as the redox potential of the water.

Let's look at the 'redox potential' closer. This redox potential can be dramatically increased by proper ionisation.

We have arrived to the theory of ionized water. We will start by exploring the bio-chemical 'background' or the reason why we get sick or (the term I like more) why the body breaks down. Remember the bank account theory? Let's see what happens when we have too much of the bad stuff. The body gets overwhelmed. This is called oxidative stress and it's a phenomenon, which results from breaking the balance between oxidative and reductive processes. Free radicals are "regulators" of all the processes taking place. The atoms are stable when their electrons are paired together (diatomic in nature, meaning they feel better when two are together). They are characterised as free radicals when they lose one of the electrons and become unpaired, they become electrically unstable triggering chain reactions or destruction within the cells.

Too many of these free radicals are a problem (mostly called ROS-reactive oxygen species, RNS- reactive nitrogen species, etc.). It has been demonstrated that these are signaling messengers showing lowered immunity, aging and gene expressions.

They have toxic effects; they can alter the redox state in the cells.

(The disturbance of ROS/RNS balance plays a pivotal role in several pathologic conditions.) At least two percent of oxygen we breathe in becomes active and will increase to twenty percent with aerobic exercise. Oxygen is stable in the air but becomes active and has a tendency to attach itself to any biological molecule, including healthy cells. It becomes a radical, has unpaired electrons or high oxidation potential so will steal electrons. Inside the body, this active radical can have a great purpose in elimination of bacteria, viruses, waste products like histamine, ammonia, phenols and indoles. Most of these are coming from the digestive track. The body's defence mechanism wants to eliminate them by releasing so called 'neutrophils.' These produce active oxygen, which is bad for us as it is extremely reactive. So, we shouldn't have too much of the bad stuff as that will create too many active radicals. If we do, however, we need to double or triple the number of antioxidants, especially our super antioxidant water. Antioxidants are substances that can protect the cells against the side effects of drugs, carcinogens and toxic radical molecules. This is why everyone is looking for good antioxidants.

"In essence, if we want to direct our lives, we must take control of our consistent actions It's not what we do once in a while that shapes our lives, but what we do consistently."

TONY ROBBINS

This is the way these consistent bad habits will make us ill. Pretty logical stuff. We should not be surprised. Now, it might be easier for you to believe how I am able to manage my health with this water.

In recent studies it has been proven that ERW, generated at the cathode during electrolysis has high pH, low dissolved oxygen and an extremely negative redox potential. It exhibits extreme scavenging potential. Because of this special property, *properly ionised water* can be the main factor in health management.

The key is that the ionisation has to be done in the right way.

Prevention means to get rid of these active free radicals. This can happen by neutralizing them. Research on the link between diet and cancer is far from complete but we know that carcinogens contribute to susceptibility to cancer. That is what carcinogen means; cancer causing! Others are called cancer fighting foods because they can stop free radical damage or oxidation. They are antioxidants. They will donate an electron where it is needed. Vitamin C and E, plus other inhibitors are reducing agents.

By supplying these needed free electrons, they block the interaction between the free radical and the normal healthy tissue.

There is no substitute for a healthy diet but it is not the best source of free electrons, I learned.

Reduced water is much more potent as it has a lot of ready to use electrons, its molecular weight is much less, it can act fast reaching all the parts of the body in a very short time. Logical, right? Digesting food takes time and is much more complicated.

We should drink a lot more and eat a lot less than we do.

I learned this the hard way.

Normal tap water or drinks in general show a positive number when their ORP [oxidation reduction potential] is measured with an ORP meter. This instrument will measure accurately the oxidation potential or respectively, the (oxidation reduction) redox potential of a fluid. Numbers

The Purple Wave

don't lie. These drinks all showing high positive numbers (+400 to +600). This shows how oxidizing they really are.

It turns out that we can drink ourselves to health or we can drink ourselves sick!

Now we are ready to look at what is going on inside the ionization chamber! The machine is hooked up to a water source, like tap for example, where minerals are present in the source water. The water goes through a special filter first and then immediately gets into the ionization chamber.

The machine is plugged into the AC outlet. The electric power in the machine is first transformed into direct current (DC) so full electrolysis can be performed. This is very important as most ionizers are not capable of producing this 230 Watts of continuous current. Due to this power the ionization begins and the water disassociates into ions.

The H+ ions are attracted to the negatively charged cathode where they are converted to molecular hydrogen (H2) according to the equation: 2e- + 2H+ –> H2. Because pH is the concentration of the H+ ions, and the amount of H+ ions are being decreased the pH increases, making the water alkaline. At this negatively charged electrode a donation of electrons take place, and the water is reduced. As soon as these H+ ions gain an electron they become neutral and highly unstable. Two of these H ions immediately pair up and hydrogen gas (H2) is formed. The cathodic water has now an abundance of hydroxide ions (OH-) to ensure high pH.

At the other electrode, the hydroxide (OH–) ions are attracted to the positive anode where they are oxidized to form H+ ions. Because pH is a measurement of the concentration of H+ ions, and the amount of H+ ions is being increased, the pH decreases, making the water acidic.

A semi-permeable ion-exchange membrane, will prevent the cathodic water (with an excess of OH- ions) and anodic water (with an excess of H+ ions) compartments from mixing together, this way producing alkaline (mild or strong) and acidic (mild or strong) water at the cathode and anode, respectively.

The big surprise of 'reduced' water is that it also becomes 'small'. How? Well, water molecules do not just float around all alone but they group together in clusters. There is no molecular bond but the attraction between the water molecules is strong enough that these molecules 'stick together'. During ionisation these clusters are broken into smaller clusters, which contain only four to six molecules and the water becomes half in size allowing this water to easily absorb into the cells. How do we know or can prove that this is happening? Some claim that NMR (Nuclear Magnetic Resonance) analysis reveals that regular/natural water consists of 10-13 molecules measuring at 133 Hz while Kangen Water® measures only at 65 Hz (at line-width at half-amplitude), which is about half the size of a normal water cluster. This is why the Japanese call it 'micro-water'. There is a bit of controversy here, as Tyler LeBaron, the well respected scientist I was mentioning before, the founder of The Molecular Hydrogen Institute states: "Although we have learned a lot of things that are not true, the structural dynamics and arrangements of liquid water remain elusive...... Physical chemists are well aware of water's mysterious nature and the many different forms of water clusters due to hydrogen bonding. Very little about water clusters in bulk phase is understood. In fact, it is considered to be one of the unsolved problems in chemistry."

What I am thinking is this; We know so little. Just because no scientific evidence exists at this time, it doesn't mean that the actual clustering theory in the water is a hoax or its non existent. Tyler my friend, you just have to research a bit further... LOL.

Our tap water after being tired and bombarded with additives becomes huge, as many as twenty-four or perhaps even more molecules stuck together.

This theory about the smaller water clusters of ionized water is not scientifically proven. Some scientist are claiming that it is not a correct conclusion at all. I am not a scientist. This is not the first or the last contradiction scientist have about something either. I can only testify to what I experienced. I know that I am experiencing powerful hydration at the cellular level, only since I am drinking Kangen water®. It is easy to drink it and many who never liked to drink water are telling me that they absolutely love this water and have no problem drinking it.

My humble opinion is that this water created in the ioniser is phenomenal but wait as I am not done with the surprises.

> **"To be prepared against surprise is to be trained. To be prepared for surprise is to be educated."**
>
> **JAMES P. CARSE**

The Purple Wave

You must admit that I did the education part, so you should be prepared and I can reveal this surprise now. The big surprise is left to the end in this "high-tech" chapter, just like in a good movie. This would be the formation of Molecular Hydrogen (H2), which is also present in Kangen Water® due to the storm we have created. This is very important as this makes Kangen Water ® different from some ionised waters.

Yes, Kangen Water® is not only alkalized and easy to absorb but also Hydrogen-Rich. While alkalinity is easy to achieve, molecular hydrogen isn't. It is hard to produce it and it is hard to keep it constant.

You need very sophisticated technology to achieve it.

Most of the time hydrogen is bonded to other atoms (see the water molecule, for example). During the storm, which goes on in the chamber, two hydrogen atoms bond together. It is, in fact, extraordinary as two Hydrogen atoms don't appear together normally in nature. It is rare. It surprised even Coanda when he saw this in the Hunza water. We can see this 'Hydrogen Gas' with the naked eye as tiny white bubbles. Another part of this hydrogen gas is dissolved and we might not be able to observe it with the naked eye. We can also hear the popping sound of this Hydrogen gas when we put an open flame near the water stream. When my water has less of these and it is 'clear' it is time to clean the plates in my machine. The two hydrogen atoms in the water molecule play a pivotal role so twice as much Hydrogen gas is produced as Oxygen gas. Nothing is a coincidence in nature! Hydrogen is the smallest and most fundamental element. This makes Molecular Hydrogen the simplest molecule in existence. Being small, light, easy and fast to penetrate, H2 will get to all parts of the body providing tremendous health benefits. We need a strong defence system in today's polluted world and H2 can provide us with this 'defence system' big time, better than anything else would. To express myself poetically,

"Not all storms come to disrupt your life, some come to clear your path."

UNKNOWN

Hydrogen was called 'water forming' by the French scientist, Antoine Lavacier. He was a noble man born in 1743 who is called the "father of modern chemistry". So, hydrogen has much more to do with water than oxygen even if it's a much smaller atom.

Hydrogen is what really turns water into water. Perhaps this is why we call the lack of water dehydration, not 'deoxydation'. (I hope I invented a new word!)

When we lack water or are dehydrated, we really lack hydrogen so dehydration is turning out to be depletion of Hydrogen in our body. So, if hydrogen deficiency is the cause, adding hydrogen is the answer, right? For decades we only heard about oxygen. Poor, tiny hydrogen was neglected ever since Henry Cavendish (1731-1810), a brilliant natural philosopher, a British chemist and physicist born in France who studied at the University of Cambridge, collected 'hydrogen' for the first time. He called hydrogen 'inflammable air'. Never underestimate small. You knew already that the 'Hydrogen bomb' is the most powerful bomb, **now you know that hydrogen gas is the most powerful antioxidant.**

Yes, there is power in a 'team' but let's not get ahead of ourselves.

The mitochondria are responsible for energy production. It will also produce free radicals as a by-product. Oxygen is also critical but part of the oxygen will turn into superoxide anions. Depending on diet, lifestyle and environmental factors, we might have too much of these free radicals, possibly more than we can handle. (Remember the bank account?) How much are you exposed to the following? Radiation, pollution, processed foods, alcohol, smoking, chemicals, heavy metals, prescription drugs, stress, mold, bacteria, viruses, lack of sleep, toxins, injuries and EMF?

In the presence of heavy metals, radiation and EMF, the cells produce the most dangerous kind of radicals called "hydroxyl" radicals. These are extremely reactive and will steal electrons from proteins, DNA and other cells hence seriously damaging them. Once they are converted, no antioxidant enzymes can neutralise them so oxidative stress is created. (We humans are not meant to be in this environment!) I am certain about this. The only way to boost our defence system against these 'modern day nightmares' is with Molecular Hydrogen.

Many companies claim that their antioxidant formula is the best but none of them have the ability of H2. Vitamin C and E are very big molecules, they need to be absorbed through the digestive system and this will slow down the process. Not in the case of H2. Each molecule,

The Purple Wave

having two hydrogen atoms, can neutralise two hydroxyl radicals. Wow. **What we have here is hydrogen 'ganging up' against the oxygen radical.**

I heard that hydrogen is three times more energy dense than gasoline. Hydrogen increases energy production and storage in the body and significantly improves fat and glucose metabolism. Wow, I like that. No wonder that I feel that sugar is not hurting me as much if I drink a good quantity of Kangen Water®.

Yes, this chapter is turning into a real action movie now but I hope you don't mind. H2, our superhero, has three amazing attributes:

1. By bonding with the free radical, it will turn it into water so we can get rid of it by peeing it out.
2. It will enhance the body's own antioxidants like glutathione, superoxide dismutase and catalase.
3. It is extremely 'smart', we call it 'selective'. This means that it will attack only the awfully bad free radicals and not the ones which the body needs to kill bacteria, for example.

So, it is safe for me to say that H2 or Molecular Hydrogen is the 'Superman' of antioxidants 'ganging up' against the 'enemy'. This is needed in today's polluted world to destroy or neutralise the effects of super oxidants like the nasty hydroxyl ion.

"The foodstuff, carbohydrate, is essentially
a packet of hydrogen, a hydrogen supplier,
a hydrogen donor, and the main event during
its combustion is the splitting off of hydrogen."

ALBERT SZENT-GYORGYI

To produce H2, a few things are needed: a constant, or continuous energy source, the conductors of the electricity (the electrolytes), solid titanium plates, Japanese precision and on and on. It makes me smile when some tell me that they are 'trying' to restructure water at home in their garage. Good luck, people. This is why simple ionisers will never make molecular hydrogen and without the hydrogen the water is not this effective.

When you go to PubMed (US Medical Library), you will find 321 articles on molecular hydrogen alone. (This number is constantly growing.)

The conclusion of this global research is this:

The therapeutic water called ERW filled with dissolved hydrogen gas formed at the cathode of the ioniser is a highly reductive water (antioxidant) and its therapeutic applications extend well beyond what is reported. In the past 50 years scientists and doctors together have never found such a powerful 'medicine' at their disposal to modify what we call "a patient's bioelectronic terrain".

It seems that everything works better when we drink this water and I think this is why. I am done with the science.

I hope this revelation of a relatively new 'scientific secret' did exceed your expectations.

"With our divine connection we are
always in touch with the
solutions we are seeking."

WAYNE DYER

Amen. I hope you appreciate the fact that the human body is brilliant and so is the fuel, which was provided for us to have abundant life here on Earth. It is amazing how we always get help from above, after we get ourselves in trouble. I am grateful!

CHAPTER 19

BIOMIMICRY

*"Nature always wears the colours
of the spirit"*

RALPH W. EMERSON

Let's do something different today. I get easily bored when I hear or see the 'same old, same old'. Let's look into revolutionary discoveries that opened new areas in biochemistry and other areas. There are great things to learn about. Many of these, of course are rooted in the marvellous 'science' of nature. **I call that Real Science.**

I love nature and everything natural. The Earth has music for those who listen. Are we listening? What is this music one can hear by praying, meditating or just having the right attitude? Here it is. It is called 'biomimicry'. Have you heard about this new trend? Biomimicry is a relatively new branch of science. Biomimicry really deserves our attention. Look at things like 'Forest Bathing' or 'Earthing'. Natural therapies are back and that is great news. It is amazing what I found as far as biomimicry goes, and these things are happening globally as we speak.

Let's look at water-based chemistry, for example. Instead of toxic solvents, science is experimenting now with simply changing the

135

structure of water leading to miraculous things. Apparently, we are not too far from creating non-toxic ink achieved with structured water. This is true biological wisdom. Nature is showing us how things should be done. The only way things should be done!

The time of man-made inventions that had devastating consequences on our health and our environment is slowly but surely coming to an end. That way of life is not sustainable. End of story.

The crazy industrial age is over, thank God, as we step into a new era called, The Ecological Age.

This makes tons of sense. Our universe provides us with millions of blueprints. It was given to us. Why not get inspired? Nature wastes nothing and recycles everything. Nature uses only a very few elements and never the toxic ones from the periodic table to sustain itself. So, let's learn wisdom from nature. Those two are in perfect harmony.

*"Never, no, never did Nature say one
thing and Wisdom say another."*

EDMUND BURKE

Most of biomimicry focuses on structure and not on 'composition'. It is observed that even the colors of the peacock are created by the structure of the feathers meeting the light and not by pigmentation or dye. This colour will not fade and it is four times brighter. It is also non-toxic, of course.

Structure is number one in my book. It is indeed. Literally and metaphorically.

*"Structure is not just a means to a solution.
It is also a principle and a passion."*

MARCEL BREUER

The Purple Wave

Look at the diamond, which has the same composition as graphite; the only difference is the structure of the matter! One is worth ten dollars, the other worth roughly one million.

What are these 'blueprints' of nature we can use? There are millions of them.

Let's take the shark for example. Did you know that the shark naturally repels all the bad bacteria from its surface? That is achieved with absolutely no chemistry, only by the special structure of its skin. Wouldn't it be nice if door knobs in hospitals had similar structure to avoid epidemics, which would eliminate the need for the toxic disinfectants used? The possibilities are endless. We just have to change our attitudes. Sustainability is a state of mind, a specific way of life. By incorporating these ideas, concepts, approaches by formal or informal education until the majority will accept and solidify them, we can become a truly eco-society.

All residents of a city or a country living sustainable lives are the foundation of a healthy community, the only community, which has a future. By these practices incorporating sustainability, common resources would be taken care of automatically. It is essential that more people would take an active role. The key to sustainability is knowledge first and then personal responsibility, implementation with commitment.

"Man cannot change a single law of nature, but can put himself into such relations to natural laws, that he can profit by them."

EDWIN GRANT CONLINK

Of course, we can profit. This is the point. It is allowed! There is 'a right way' of doing thigs to the contrary of popular belief. We just have to love nature and the Creator of nature more than we love money! There are so many examples that you won't have enough time to listen to all of them if you look up Biomimicry. My favorite example, of course, is Kangen Water®. No chemical change. Kangen Water® only has structural changes inspired by nature's blueprint. This is the closest we can come to Nature's water at this time. In this sense using a Kangen machine is a responsibility towards our environment.

We must create conditions for life, not disaster. This is my main message to you. What good is killing the bad bacteria if we kill the good bacteria at the same time? Why do we kill our healthy cells with cancer 'treatments'? Cancer is not the tumour. The tumour is only the symptom. Your oncologist doesn't understand this. What's tragic is that many people trust these blinded professionals who are paid to be blind. One hundred years from now, the world will be puzzled; "How on Earth did those poor people expect to get better, injecting poisons into their veins!?"

Healthy people get really ill or die from radiation. How is that good for the ill whose health is already compromised? Please call me if you know the answer...

We have to smarten up very fast because millions are dying from irresponsible, unethical and ineffective 'interventions' or just plain, stupid ideas. Millions are getting diabetes and other chronic conditions from drinking fruit juices or colored sugary drinks, instead of water. To eat the fruit in its natural state together with all the fibre is healthy. To destroy that fibre and drink the fruit instead of water has consequences as the fruit juice is natural but the way we eat and prepare food is also important. In this case, the body won't be able to handle all that sugar coming into the blood stream too fast in over concentrated quantity, without any fibre. There is a reason why the fruit has fibre. Nature doesn't make mistakes. Pay attention to details. Eat fruit as much as you like, just don't try to replace water with it because that is just plain stupid! Many avoid fruits (the best food we have and I eat tons of it) because they don't understand that it is the lack of water, lack of exercise and what not and not the fruit, which is causing diabetes and other issues.

"In a major matter, no details are too small."

JEAN F. PAUL de GONDI

"The truth of the story lies in the details."

PAUL AUSTER

The Purple Wave

Ladies and Gentleman: The science behind the technology of the Kangen® machine is 50 years ahead of what we call biomimicry today. The water of the Hunzas inspired a big group of scientists who contributed in creating this superior quality water. I consider Kangen Water® an extremely successful method of mimicking nature. Enagic® is well ahead of the curve and this is why we are having a hard time with closed-minded people. By having a machine in every house we can instantly eliminate the huge issue of plastic bottles. It is just a matter of time. We all should wake up to this new reality!

Soft drinks, marketed beverages and everything packaged in plastic, which is not found in nature has turned out to be a disaster. They cause addictions and they ruin our health. **So, can this brilliant product be the next trend defining the modern Eco-kitchen?**

You bet. The need is tremendous. The distraction caused by non reusable plastic bottles and containers has to stop! These can't be part of our environment as they are not organic in nature.

I love Da Vinci's unparalleled wisdom:

"Those who are inspired by a model other than Nature, labor in vain."

LEONARDO DA VINCI

Isn't that the truth? A truth, which has stood the test of time. **I call that the Real Truth.**

CHAPTER 20

SCAM ARTISTS

"So, we should no longer be children, tossed about as by waves and carried here and there by every wind of teaching, by means of trickery of man, by means of cunning in deceptive schemes."

EPHESIANS 4.14

Who is watching, who is responsible? Bottled water defined as 'food' under federal regulation is under the authority of the FDA (Food and Drug Administration) in the USA, or Health Canada, in Canada. The EPA (Environmental Protection Agency) is an old collaboration between the USA and Canada who regulates our tap water, under stricter standards. Thus, bottled water is less clean and safe than tap water. We all know how the FDA operates. Huge holes exist in the regulatory fabric of bottled waters. Water companies do not always comply with standardized contamination levels.

Man-made tricks and deceptive schemes will never work when it comes to the nutrition of humans or animals for that matter. Look at the dog food industry! Everyone who I know is switching from dog 'food' to other alternatives because the poor animals are also suffering and dying

The Purple Wave

from cancer. Another industry invented by scam artists! Dogs, cats and horses also can be helped Kangen Water®. They are drinking water filled with chemicals such as chorine and other additives, which are harmful in the long run.

Altering the chemistry of water, by adding stuff like baking soda, additives, chlorine, fluoride or any other stuff is causing serious problems. **This water will not be functional. This is the main reason 95 percent of us are chronically dehydrated, I think.**

"All the symptoms of aging are in one way or another accompanied by a slow dehydration of our vital tissues associated with free radical damage," says, Dr. Flanagan, a famous M.D. from the United States. He received the Scientist of the Year award in 1997. He was a child prodigy with an intense interest in both electronics and biochemistry and who met Dr. Coanda when he was only 17-years-old.

Dehydration is becoming a serious issue as time goes by. Why is that? I believe that this new habit of people replacing water with marketed drinks, which has the exact opposite effect and further dehydrates the body, are responsible.

Let's look a bit closer at the biggest scam in history, a scam that is quietly causing unprecedented damage when it comes to health. **This whole industry is nonsense. A classic example of clever marketing is the brainwashing of people for the last five decades - especially children - of marketed drinks being good for consumers.**

These drinks are offered to the public everywhere; they are called 'the new cigarettes' by some as they are planted carefully at eye level for kids and are advertised just like cigarettes were 50 years ago. They are causing serious addictions. At the beginning, when they were first developed, kids were offered one drink on their birthday or at the New Year's party, maybe. Lately people replaced water with them as they are sold at every corner store and restaurant, every vending machine or gas station. Thankfully, I never liked such drinks, so addiction wasn't an issue for me but two of my family members got hooked on these processed beverages. We tried many ways to get them off but nothing worked. Thanks to Kangen Water®, they had no problem quitting all sodas in about two weeks.

"The more hidden the venom,
the more dangerous it is."

MARGUERITE DE VALOIS

A Natural Resources Defense Council study found that: "Eighteen of the 103 bottled water brands tested contained more bacteria than allowed under legal microbiological-purity standards." Many brands also tested positive for the presence of synthetic chemicals, industrial chemicals, etc. In addition, bottled water industries are not required to test for cryptosporidium, a chlorine-resistant protozoan that infected more than 400,000 Milwaukee residents in 1993.

Now you know. **Marketed drinks should not be used instead of water.** I call them 'Satan in a bottle'. I know, I know ... I am nasty; but wait until you see how horrible the people who market these drinks are. To sell it to you, they were named 'soft' drinks. They are called soft with a purpose. Soft you see, never hurts. Soft is desirable. It is soft, not like evil, hard liqueur. The truth is, soft drinks are much worse than pure alcohol and just as addictive, if not more; but all people hear is that they are 'soft'. Many are fooled by the energising power of energy drinks but that is fake energy, made with tons of sugar, artificial sweeteners which are neurotoxins that are much worse than natural sugar (which is bad and addictive enough). A well thought out scam.

This is what I call a 'landmine' for the unsuspecting one.

Hopefully you will read my upcoming book called, "ARE YOU SINKING? HERE COMES A BOAT! ". In this book, I will present the hidden landmines of modern society, in greater detail.

It took about thirty years until people realized they needed to supplement with vitamins and anti-oxidants as the food we eat has less and less nutritional value. I am wondering how long it will take to get this one. The only way to get away from marketed drinks is to drink living water, a healthy and natural alternative. Nowadays, you hear the command: Drink eight to ten glasses of water a day, especially if you do physical activity. Really everyone should - but no one tells you where to find the water you should be drinking. Perhaps a real revolution is needed, and definitely some education is needed in this regard!

Bottled water companies as they are not under the same accountability standards as municipal water systems, provide a significantly lower quality of water than your tap. They also enjoy a loophole or two. They set up shops in different states and provinces diminishing the local water supply and selling processed tap water back to residents at a huge mark up, with no rules! How much longer are we going to be silent about this crime?

The Purple Wave

*"Energy drinks like Red Bull may give you wings
for the moment, but in time it takes away
your basic physical & mental wellness
and leads to disastrous psychiatric
and physiological conditions."*

ABHIJIT NASCAR

Are you using any of these? How about your family members? They might need your help. Without good water they will never be able to get rid of their addiction to these.

CHAPTER 21

MODERN DAY HERO

"The prudent see only the difficulties, the bold only the advantages of a great enterprise; the HERO sees both, diminishes the former and makes the latter preponderate, and so conquers."

JOHANN KASPAR LAVATER

Many contributed to the fulfillment of Albert Szent-Gyorgyi's prediction, *"Who can change the structure of the water in the living systems, will change the world!"* One hero I want to mention is *Dr. YOSHIAKI MATSUO, PH.D.* of course, who is the actual inventor of the ioniser. He is the cause of a real *'Water Boom'*, not the bottling companies. They caused a water crisis. Soon after this discovery, in 1965, *"The Ministry of Health and Welfare of Japan announced that micro water is superior to any antioxidant diet and it can prevent fermentation of intestinal microbes."* This micro water compared to any water available today, anywhere around the globe, is beyond comparison because of the very high Oxidation Reduction Potential, which makes it a free radical scavenger.

Thus, the moto, "Change your water, change your life® is not a marketing slogan, but rather a real solution to change people's health!

How did Kangen Water® appear on the 'world stage' or today's global market? Would you like to know this part of the story? It is quite interesting. Please read the quote under the title of this chapter once again as it describes our hero with 100 percent accuracy.

The person who made this possible and therefore 'conquered the world' isn't a famous doctor with impressive credentials or a scientist who is part of the system but a humble man from a small island. He struggled a lot in his life and now, with the help of others like myself is making the world a much better and happier place. Mr. Ohshiro recognised the importance of this idea, this technology created by his co-patriot. Yes, this tool was brought to humanity forty-five years ago by a man called Hironari Ohshiro, born on March 17, 1941 in Okinawa, Japan. Coming from a poor family, he had a hard life and he lost most of his siblings to malaria. He is rightfully considered a modern-day hero.

As far as I am concerned, the unbelievable, but true story of David and Goliath is repeated once again by Mr. 'O', as we call him. Did you know that this biblical story was studied in great depth by expert scholars who found that the reason David succeeded in killing Goliath was not because of his position, fame, or title? Not even because of his physical strength. Obviously, there were many greater and more accomplished warriors in the army of Israel but because he had a special tool and a skill he had mastered. He understood where to hit a person to instantly kill him. This was his secret besides having extraordinary courage, which only people with faith have.

Likewise, our hero, Mr. 'O' approaching 80 now, the kindest man walking on Earth, recognised and grabbed a tremendous tool that had the potential to change the world. The technology was ready, but someone with courage, faith and exceptional morals needed to bring it to the masses. Mr. 'O' did not give up until he succeeded and he is still going strong. The unthinkable happened;

The secret got out and now, it appears in front of you in bold print.

What is your opinion about this? Are you just a bit excited or do you need some water to help you comprehend this? This might sound nasty but I assure you that is not my intention. We find that people's brains are often so dehydrated and acidic that comprehension or even making good decisions can be a challenge or impossible. I feel horrible for people in that situation. Some people's thinking is improved as soon as they start drinking and this happens in as fast as two weeks. Anyhow, now many of us know that **Japanese scientists have mastered a technology that has an unprecedented potential to help humanity.**

This technology, however, had to be tried on real people. It wasn't meant to be a lab experiment. This is why only now, after decades of human consumption, we know what it does. Wow!

I am thrilled that I am alive today. All I feel is gratefulness.... tremendous amounts of gratefulness.

"Enjoy the little things, for one day
you may look back and realize
they were the big things."

ROBERT BRAULT

Today's 'Goliath', Big Pharma, is very strong. We need as many little "Davids" as we can find. We need people like you to share this information with others.

Did you lose a loved one, prematurely? When I lost my parents, the guilt I felt because I couldn't do anything for them almost killed me. Do you know anyone who is having health issues? With this ultimate tool, we have an opportunity to make a difference in a world which seems to be out of control. You don't have to be a chemist or a rocket scientist to make a difference! This machine, which is certified as a medical device in Japan, makes it possible for people in big cities and small places to have access to water that is just as healthy and pure as the glacier waters of the Himalayas.

This is big news! As soon as this becomes common, we will substantially expand the 'BLUE ZONES'!

On my recent trip to Toronto, people I talked to on the plane, on buses and in restaurants told me that they are looking for a 'solution' for drinking water. This tells me that people slowly but surely are waking up to a new reality. What a tremendous problem people are facing in polluted cities right now. In British Columbia's 2018 forest fire season when we had over 500 fires around us, the smoke not only got really scary, but straight out choking. My lungs never experienced anything like this before and I was not alone with this problem. Drinking a lot from my water absolutely saved my life. The extra oxygen and hydrogen I successfully shovelled down my throat made breathing much easier and calmed me down. I probably avoided a few panic attacks. It felt like there was nowhere to go. We were traveling one heavy smoky day through the mountains and it wasn't going well for either of us. As you are probably suspecting, we did survive. What a relief and help this was for us, when so many ended up ill and/or hospitalized.

> *"Anyone who can solve the problems of water will be worthy of two Noble Prizes-one for peace and one for science."*
>
> *J.F. KENNEDY*

I definitely agree with J.F.K. Two or more Nobel Prizes, but more importantly the recognition and the respect of humanity.

The technology to produce good, living water once again is introduced now to many different countries around the world. Mr. 'O', our hero is achieving his dream to make the world a better place and all of us who recognise this can and will benefit. This is as good as it gets.

Over 1,000 years ago, natural water had this quality and purity, experts are saying.

There are many modern-day heroes who dedicate their lives to repairing and undoing the damages from different disasters all around the world. There are many people who fight the good fight... I love heroes.

> *"Heroism feels and never reasons, and therefore, is always right."*
>
> *UNKNOWN*

CHAPTER 22

DEATH TO POISONS!

"The poison of selfishness
destroys the world."

CATHRINE OF SIENA

We are exposed to never-before-seen amounts of poison. We must live with man-made chemicals, endocrine disruptors, hormone disruptors and more. Every day tons of toxic matter are used all around us, destroying the purity and quality of our food and water supply. I feel sorry for pregnant women as birth defects are also on the rise. Everything, we adults, are exposed to is much more dangerous for new-born babies who's immune system is not developed just yet.

For the first time in 200 years children will not live as long as their parents. We are going backwards!

Kangen Water®, an eco-friendly and cost-effective solution is here, yet some are trying to stop it from getting well known by the masses by calling it a scam, a pyramid scheme, a magic trick or simply 'just-water', water which has no meaning or benefits to anyone. They are threatened. It's not hard to understand how worried they might be jeopardizing the sales of these poisonous chemicals.

The Purple Wave

Chemicals for a few decades took over the world. They turned that industry into a money-making machine. These chemicals are not good for anyone, not even for the makers but they keep producing them, because they are blinded by profits. We, Kangen Water® users, you see, save about $200 plus monthly on average by replacing household chemicals, bottled water, beverages, skin care products and much more with the different grades of water that we are able to access from the technology. There are seven different grades or five kinds of water the machine produces. The 8.5, 9.0 and 9.5 pH waters are typically for drinking while more acidic or more alkaline ones are used for many different purposes. This is the reason why I like to say that all the waters from the machine are not only blue and purple, but also green - green in every sense of the word. The whole machine is so environmentally friendly that our ecological footprint is substantially reduced when we use it to its full extent compared to the traditional way of doing things. Our carbon footprint, water footprint, health care cost and our economy are all affected in a positive way by the use of the Kangen® machine. By Wikipedia, a 'carbon footprint' is historically defined as the total emissions caused by an individual, event, organization, or product, expressed as carbon dioxide equivalent.

This would be such progress from the environmental standpoint as well as from the medical prospective that its use should be mandated by law, as far as I am concerned. Our modern society would benefit tremendously from this innovation and the lifestyle which comes with it. Brand new industries could be developed and money still could be made by shifting to a new way of thinking with the best interest of our environment in perspective. The direction must change! Simple.

"You cannot get through a single day without having an impact on the world around you. What you do makes a difference, and you have to decide what kind of impact you want to make."

JANE GOODALL

We decided. Many of us replaced prescription pills and substantially reduced the amount of supplements we are taking when we started drinking this water! We are not against progress. We are for real progress. Progress, which makes things better and makes sense.

This is what happened to Roger, mentioned earlier, a man who I admire and whose story should be heard by the nations. He was taking lots a different medications for years and once he started on Kangen Water® they got gradually 'replaced'. Imagine, one person alone has saved over $80,000 in tax payers' money if not more by now. Marvelous, don't you think so? I mentioned it to you before; this water makes a lot of sense and solves a lot of problems.

To be truly green doesn't happen often with technology. Enagic® has done it successfully and realistically, however. We are lifting a heavy burden when we get rid of plastic bottles and numerous chemicals.

I call this a miracle, a blessing and simply amazing. Again, wining and whimpering about the environment wont help the environment. Doing something like changing our lifestyles will.

> *"Environmental pollution is an 'incurable disease'. It can only be prevented."*
>
> **BARRY COMMOVER**

In beautiful British Columbia, we have stores now where absolutely everything we should use for skin care, hair care and such is made of natural raw materials. It is more expensive, but in the long run, this natural lifestyle will be cheaper. From a shampoo bar, which doesn't need a plastic bottle to natural shaving cream there is everything one might use or need. From candles to essential oils, you can stay natural. There are solutions, many of them. It is only a matter of people using them.

We have to maintain the right balance in our lifestyle which will help to maintain homeostasis. Kangen Water® makes it easy to achieve that.

Homeostasis means bio-chemical and electrical balance.

Why do we want to do that? Because when our body gets to this 'stage of balance' it will heal itself. We will prevent a breakdown of our immune system. We can have a brain that will work as long as our body

The Purple Wave

will and a body that will work as long as our brain is intact. We don't have to live in fear thinking that we will be the next victim of a stroke. Many people are surprised when they develop blood clots and have no idea that the prescription pills they are taking are causing those!

It is extremely beneficial to downsize and simplify. I did. Less stress means a better and longer life. Let's invest in our family's future. Your child needs good water more than the latest smart phone or video game. Let's think before we spend our hard-earned money.

I don't have a magic camera to show you what is happening inside the body when we drink this 're-structured' water but we are able to see with a proper microscope what happens to the blood and that is mind-blowing. By thinning the blood naturally as it should be, for example, we can get our blood pressure under control with water. Bring plenty of oxygen to the blood by water. Clean your colon with water. I did. I also maximised or at least improved my brain function with water. Simple common sense.

> *"My rhymes are like stop watches,*
> *interstate cops*
> *and blood clots,*
> *my point is your flow gets stopped."*
>
> **Talib Kweli**

Blood clots or strokes are not something I would joke about.

The best tool I have ever seen to prevent a stroke or two or three is Kangen Water® and you can take that to the bank! Water is a natural blood thinner!

Not long ago I came across a documentary about professional bakers in Austria. They made a discovery, which spread like wildfire all over Europe. The bakers realised that the dough they used to make bread was not working as it should, not because of the quality of the flour or the yeast, but because the water they used was 'dead'. It had no power to do its job any longer and so the bread didn't rise properly. Can you do your job when you are tired? Anyhow, they came up with this marvellous idea, a common sense idea I would say. They revitalised the water by using huge ioniser machinery and now they say that since they have been making bread with 'living' water, they can use substantially less yeast, no chemicals and no additives, yet the bread smells amazing, tastes better, has a thinner crust, is softer and it lasts longer. I love success stories. I actually know people who get angry or frustrated as soon as they hear about someone's success. Let's get you away from them.

Cheer up! Having all this info you can get revitalized! I hope you are not afraid of living life to the fullest. In that case, avoid our water. With all seriousness, don't you find this kind of important? The endless adding of chemicals is not the answer for bakers. Why would it be for us, human beings?

People are always looking and spending like crazy for skin and hair care (some corporations might bring me to Court for this) because they don't realise that it is the water which needs to be changed, not the products they are using. **The 'processed water' is what makes your hair look ugly or impossible to handle, not necessarily your shampoo!**

I recently stayed a whole month in Toronto and my hair was absolutely horrible, looked dull and lifeless as I was showering with chlorinated water. There was nothing I could do to make it better. As soon as I returned home and used my 'ANESPA' shower unit with 6 pH water, chlorine free, my hair was shiny and beautiful again, washed with the same soap I always use, with no conditioner or any other product. Chlorinated water doesn't only kill rats, it destroys everything that has life. Everyone needs chlorine free water in their bathroom, not only in the kitchen.

> *"The governments weaponize toxins that the masses are routinely exposed to, and then denies the known toxicity of them."*
>
> **STEVEN MAGEE**

We very much need the armor of God in our spiritual lives; however, we also need this 'armor' for our physical wellbeing and survival. Now, after people have been poisoned by 'safe' ink, we are seeing more tattoo removing studios. Finally, something is changing. I have a great feeling

The Purple Wave

about the future in this regard. Many are expressing great concerns regarding our environment. There are new ideas and initiatives in almost every country, all around the globe. The negative media never mentions these, so I thought, I should mention it.

I also learned on this journey that with all the obsession we have with our diets today, food is only twenty-five percent of the diet puzzle. 75 percent is what we are drinking. Again, the majority do not know about the 75 percent, which is the fluid our cells are bathing in and where all chemical reactions take place. Dr. Colbert calls water "the first and most important pillar of health". He is right as the 75 percent is so powerful that in many cases it will take care of 'the twenty-five percent'. Now, because I can detox and balance myself right away with my special water, I can eat almost anything I like (I only like and tolerate chemical or preservative free natural foods as I said it before.) or even have a glass of wine. I have not been able to do that for years.

We need good fat, lots of water, organic raw nutrients and not aluminium, poisons, neurotoxins, heavy metals, synthetic pills for the proper functioning of our brain and body.

"Everything is toxic. That's the point.
You can't avoid toxins. Thinking that
you can, is just another symptom of
the toxic overload stages."

JANE SMIL

This was before the Kangen® machine. The future suddenly became brighter. Get this as this is huge. The oxidised water from the anode of the Kangen® machine has a redox potential around +1000. This Hyperoxidized Water is another exciting thing I have come across. This is biomimicry at its best. This water called Hypochlorous acid (HOCl) is not only a very powerful oxidizing agent, which rapidly kills things like MRSA or STAPH, but also has great potential when we apply it to the field of agriculture. Imagine an agent, which kills fungi and other plant diseases and it's not toxic, at all. Workers in agriculture could use this water without protective equipment as there is no danger of poisoning or respiratory damage. You can spray this water into your eyes and it won't hurt you. It won't hurt anything living but the bad bacteria as its not chemical acid. It won't hurt people when we eat the blueberries and fruits. We can forget all about carcinogens like the herbicides used today. There will be no accumulation of toxic stuff in the ground! The possibilities for a better, eco-friendly future are endless. I am really excited about this. So are the marijuana growers. They are buying industrial size Kangen machines, as the water makes a huge difference in the lives of the plants. These marijuana plants sadly look much better than many dried out humans I meet. I wish I could help everyone, but of course that is not the case.

CHAPTER 23

PEE, STRUCTURE AND OTHER MIRACLES

"Miracles happen every day; change your perception of what a miracle is, and you will see them all around you."

BON JOVI

Some people's perception of miracles sucks. I agree, that's why they never see any. I have seen many recoveries which can be considered miracles. We, the users of this water, are not hypocrites. We are all using it and have been every day for years. We are thriving because of it in an otherwise unhealthy environment and those of us who care, we want the same for everyone.

The only 'bad news' (at least for some), that should be mentioned perhaps, is that if we drink more water we are going to pee more. What a miracle peeing is. As far as I know, it wasn't announced yet, not on the world wide web, not on the news, or anywhere else that people can stop peeing just because everyone is stuck in traffic, is busy, lazy or something. I am actually suspecting that peeing is one of those eternal laws I mentioned before. Those who have to pee, don't want to pee. Ask someone who is not able to pee! They would love to pee but they have to use a catheter or they are on dialysis.

So, the natural cycle, the way the body cleans and protects itself is by drinking water and then peeing. Drinking and peeing is a beautiful thing. It is a necessary one. In the case of Kangen Water®, the more we pee, the happier we get. I would say, let's drink to that, at least, until the politicians change the law, regarding this 'privilege'. Why I am saying this? Believe it or not, some people don't even want to pee. They will find an excuse why they can't, so they want to control this aspect of their lives. This is a sad situation. I don't really want to comment on this. I don't even know what to say, I am speechless and I prefer to stay in a good mood. Anger or frustration will destroy the 'structure 'of the cell water, remember? Water is sensitive to feelings and moods, attitudes or negative energy.

We need to get back to our beautiful subject: health and happiness, through water, the most amazing substance on Earth.

As a summary, the unique characteristics of ERW are: Molecular Hydrogen - which turns it into the most powerful antioxidant, the negative charge [-300 to - 800 mV], a bio-available structure and the high pH [8.5 -9.5]. All these will work *together* to recharge your batteries, and to hydrate you at the cellular level. I personally have never seen anything this powerful, this therapeutic.

85 percent of the populous is magnesium deficient and that affects the heart along with the rest of the muscles besides the many other functions it has. Nothing is added to Kangen Water®, no hidden, inorganic minerals in the filter or some place else and it is loaded with Magnesium which is recognized by the body. Most ionizer companies do add minerals. They however don't want you to know that so they usually hide it in the filter. It is very easy to find that 'trick' by simply adding the pH value of the two waters coming out at the two hoses. If the total number is over fourteen, then the water has been tampered with an 'additive', which is inorganic. In case of the Kangen Water®, all health benefits are simply the result of electrolysis, which is in fact electrical chemistry, a totally different method. Finally, no chemicals. Yay! This fact alone is huge and deserves our admiration.

Inorganic minerals are not bioavailable, says Dr. Peggy Parker. "When we consume too many inorganic minerals, they create crystalline structures in the tissues of the body, which tend to gather wherever the weakest organs or systems are so some people will get kidney stones, gall

The Purple Wave

stones, arthritis, gout, bone spurs, hardening of the arteries, cataracts... while people may not experience bad health immediately overtime they build up and create some serious health problems." I had gall stones at age thirty-three and kidney stones at age 50, probably because I was taking tons of calcium pills and calcium intravenously since age eighteen. My daughter, myself and a few others I know got rid of kidney stones, not long after they switched to Kangen Water®. I see it often how this amazing water works in everyday life because we share hundreds of gallons. My compromised and genetically weak liver in particular is enjoying this naturally clean water.

The world-famous scientist, Ray Kurzweil, is another huge fan of ERW. He has credibility and respect in the scientific community. An inventor himself, he answers the skeptics by drinking ten glasses of restructured water every day. He is the inventor of the first print-to-speech reading machine for the blind, the first text-to-speech synthesizer, the first music synthesizer capable of recreating the grand piano and other instruments and much more. He was born in New York City in 1948. He is often called by nick names like 'the restless genius', or 'the ultimate thinking machine.'

Kangen Water® is different from other ionised waters as they simply don't have the power to make ionisation real.

To do that, a minimum of 230 Watts of power is required. When you read the paperwork, make sure to look into the original information from the manufacturer. Often, different wholesalers try to manipulate people with fake documentation. Unfortunate, but we have seen it!

Those who become experts on Google in 'twenty minutes' can easily fall into the hands of con artists.

It is not only the structure of the water but the unique structure of the compensation plan that makes Enagic different from all other companies.

Enagic® is a human based network, in a formation of 'direct selling' and not multi level (MLM) in its structure.

This special, patented compensation plan is what makes Enagic® the envy of the business world.

Different structures give different results. I have to use the example of 'a plastic bag'. Once I had the chance to talk to a chemist and he tried to explain it to me how margarine (some eat that stuff) has the same components as a plastic bag with only a tiny difference in it's structure. Since then, I remember that structure is really important. For how many years have you been eating plastic bags? I never bought into 'margarine' but I did buy into refined sugar years ago until I became addicted.

It is amazing what we can achieve with the right structure.

"An individual cannot be considered entirely sane if he is wholly ignorant of scientific method and structure of nature and so retains primitive semantic reactions."

— *Alfred Korzybski*

We saw how structured water works so much better than bulk water. Wait until you see our pay system. What most people desire is fair pay. That is hard or maybe even impossible to achieve with traditional MLM. Enagic® has a fair pay plan, thanks to it's 'eight-point' system. What that means is that if you don't work, you won't get paid. More you work, more you will get paid. Simple. Every effort to the smallest details is taken care of by this unique compensation system. There are all sorts of educational bonuses (when we train and mentor other distributors) which I am not going to explain here. To see all this in detail, please go to YouTube and look for our compensation plan. It's not a secret. Every distributor at Enagic® has to work hard to achieve success and as long as it is based on the person's own efforts and not luck or other people's hard work, it makes it a fair system.

"Hard work is a 'prison sentence' only if it does not have meaning..."

MALCOLM GLADWELL

Oh, people getting better is extremely meaningful to me. Another big advantage for the new consumer is our 'water share'. This is one of the reasons why this machine is not sold at stores. We want you to have a free (no obligation) trial and actually drink the water long enough so that

The Purple Wave

you feel the benefits before you buy. Have you ever bought something you regret or that didn't work? I did. Mr. Ohshiro chose human based marketing for this reason. Water sharing in neighborhoods or in families could not be done if the machine was sold in stores. I don't know about another company which lets you try the water for any length of time. We can easily guess why. Try to find another company like Enagic® with offices and service centres all around the world. It doesn't exist!

I have to share with you a 'structure story' from 1986 at the International Symposium on Cancer. The idea of 'Molecular water environment theory' was discussed in details at this symposium. The theory is based on the scientific discovery that a greater structure of water is surrounding healthy DNA cells than cancerous cells. Research indicates that the way water molecules are organised around DNA is an indication of aging and disease. I find this more than interesting. It tells me that I really should believe the 'structure theory'.

I know it's true because the cancer industry would not be threatened by it if it wasn't significant and true. It is revolting but not surprising that since 1986, the Cancer Society is still mute about the structure of cell water but it makes sense. Just imagine the money lost, if everyone knew about this mind-blowing information. How would they make money? Are you one of those 'good hearted' people who keep donating to those crooks?

"If you want to understand function, study structure."

FRANCIS CRICK

Dear friends, **we have to get the knowledge and a machine in every household and instead of marching for the 'cure' (which of course will never happen), let's stop the cause!** Am I making sense?

Now, we need to mention this; Sugar! Today, we know about the negative effects of sugar. The story of sugar is written in books. I found one of them. I came across this book seventeen years ago. This well written and very informative book (sorry I can't remember the title) was written 120 years ago and there was a prediction in it. Already then, the industry knew how detrimental it would be for people, however, the 'process' was never stopped. So, the effects of sugar were well known for many decades and this important information was suppressed. The sugar industry as a whole is considered one of history's worst conspiracies against the masses. Sugar feeds cancer. Sugar is still pushed. Every corner store and gas station (many placed intentionally near schools) is filled with sugar up to the ceiling!

> **"The three most harmful addictions are heroin, sugar and a monthly salary."**
>
> **NASSIM N. TALEB**

I consider Kangen Water® a new tool in dealing with sugar. The more I drink, the less harm I experience. It is noticeable how the water breaks down the sugar and helps with the elimination of it. I find this amazing.

The structure of the water in an infant's body is undeniably greater than in the body of an adult. The population should take full advantage of this information. We should all continue to learn, especially doctors.

Some people tell me that they have to 'ask their doctor' before they start drinking better quality water. This would be okay, if the doctor is familiar with natural, alternative, water as a blood thinner, etc., but often this is not the case. Often those who should know the facts are not knowledgeable about water.

I have a problem with health professionals who won't even look into or study ionised water before they form an opinion.

> **"The art of healing comes from nature and not the physician. Therefore, the physician must start from nature, with an open mind."**
>
> **PARACELSUS**

I don't want to rely on testimonials or claims no matter how amazing they are. We have facts thanks to a study conducted by Dr. Horst Filtzer,

The Purple Wave

an eminent cardiovascular surgeon in the USA who lives in Arizona. He is the former Chief of Surgery of Cambridge Hospital and a well-respected and well-known Harvard graduate Dr. Filtzer is part of the group of pioneer cardiovascular surgeons who first implanted the 'Stent', into the heart. The stent is a small mesh tube used quite often now to enlarge narrow arteries. Because of this idea, people with narrowed arteries do not need bypass surgeries any longer. Fred, my husband has two of these placed in his arteries. Isn't it spectacular what some doctors can come up with? Dr. Filtzer is a very humble and a very friendly man. He and I had a long, interesting conversation in a bar in Vegas while attending a conference and the funny thing was that we were both drinking Kangen Water®, not alcohol. Believe it or not we still had a great time. I would dare to say that we probably got 'high' on water.

Dr. Filtzer's next 'adventure' is to do more scientific studies with Kangen Water®; phase two is in the making. The first phase, which was conducted between 2014 and 2016 resulted in a book called: *"Scientific Study Results on the Benefits of Kangen Water® in the Human Tissue Cultures and Living Human Volunteers"*. The whole study was done in an independent and accredited lab, of course, and the conclusions are simple, clear, scientific and factual. We don't have to rely on claims, we got facts!

Here are the Facts, according to Dr. Filtzer's study: Kangen Water® from an SD501® made by Enagic® in Osaka, Japan, has amazingly beneficial effects on humans.

These are not limited to, but include:

- Increased red cell production
- Increased oxygen delivery and carbon dioxide removal (I love this!)
- Improved function of the cellular engine
- Increased production of platelets
- Improved stress induced damage repair
- Significant reduction of inflammation
- Improved recovery from injury and oxidation!
- Improved cellular metabolism and enhanced energy production in the presence of glucose.

In general, Kangen Water® has only positive effects on the mitochondria responsible for the breakdown of sugars. It is simple and logical. I hope that you wont take this significant study lightly. You can use it! You can put it in practice...

People's lives are made better daily.

We have seen significant results with some people's kidney functions.

None of the waters made by other ionizers have been used in real medical studies on humans, except Kangen water.®Be aware! "Kangen" is a trademarked name, so it's use by other companies except 'Enagic' is illegal.

I don't like to be a 'lab rat'. Yes, they make, they claim and they sell these ionizers but no one knows what kind of materials they use, what is leeching into the water, etc. Just saying...

It was reassuring for me to see the "increased production of platelets" from this study, proven in everyday life. We could help an eight-year-old boy about two years ago. His life was endangered by the lack of platelets in his blood. Medical professionals had no answer for him. I knew about his situation through the great grandmother who was our client. When I read the study results, I showed the book to the parents. They made an effort and got a machine. After a few months of drinking the water, the little boy's platelet count and his blood are completely normal. The parents are so happy ... their happiness brought them a second child. I am so happy for them. What a story. Have you realised yet what Dr. Batman and I realised? These kids are not really ill, they are often dehydrated to a point of no return and at times they die, or they are misdiagnosed before the root cause is found.

The population is tired. Water is the largest single source of energy. This alone should suggest to all that the problem might be dehydration. The skeptic will not look at water. After all, water is just water. It doesn't come with a name like 7 UP, which will bring you 7 x 7 'down', definitely not 'up'. Yes, you will need about 42 glasses of Kangen Water® to neutralise one glass of soda. I told you that advertisers are very clever. They know how to fool you, yet you think that Enagic® distributors are fooling people. Now you know!

I witnessed how this water became the new symbol of love for people. Why? When we share water, we are actually sharing love and compassion. I sincerely believe that you can't love yourself, your family or the environment and not embrace this. This doesn't mean that there are no negative reports out there but that is only on Google. We know that those reviews are only opinions and not facts. What you must know is that Google is filled with information by advertisers who pay for the platform. Once they pay, they can say whatever they want. Form your own opinion, don't let advertisers mess with your mind.

"The most courageous act is still to think for yourself..."

COCO CHANEL

The better something is, the more it is attacked. Some people can't comprehend that. Remember Jesus? Could he be better than he was? Could he have been attacked more viciously? Both answers are 'no', of course. Can water get better than Kangen Water®? Not likely! Nothing happened in forty-five years. The so-called 'mesh' technology won't do it. There is not enough surface area, no matter how many plates are used to do the job properly. How do you clean mesh? I am convinced that cleaning mesh is not possible. What do you do when something with holes gets dirty and moldy from water? You throw it out! So, how long will it take for your mesh plated ioniser to become moldy and dirty? What do you think? Could you ever clean your sticky tub mat full with tiny holes after it got moldy or would you have to throw it out?

Now you know why the good old SD501 is attacked by some who want to sell you something else. All they can say is 'old technology'! Yes, it is and it's working. Comparing an ionizer to a Kangen® machine is like comparing apples with oranges.

Water generating systems, filters or any other devices are not regulated in Canada. The population has no idea. Anything goes. Everything can be sold. Health Canada is "recommending" water generating devices which are certified by 'health standards'! I only know one. I also know that now other companies are trying to get different certifications so they can sell better but who is really the 'authority'? Is it someone who is paid off or is it someone who wants to make money? We know that they are paying celebrities to endorse their products.

Regular ionisers are not capable of making 2.5 and 11.5 pH waters, both of which are needed in a household for different reasons. To produce that low acidity and that high alkalinity, you need to add extra sodium and extra chloride to the water. The Kangen® machine is the only one which has a 'solution tank' in order to add this salt solution to the water. The machine is so 'smart' that it will 'divide' this enhancer and use the Sodium to make the 11.5 pH and the Chloride to make 2.5 pH waters. This feature of the machine is the envy of the industry!

The only negative you will find about the Kangen machine is by people who never used it. How can you have an opinion about something you have never tried? Are those competent people? You decide. Find one person who has used Kangen Water® for years and is not happy with it. You won't find such a person. Ninety percent of people buy this product only for personal use so they are not selling it. Why would they still say great things about it and share their testimony?

I call this simply Compassion.

> ### *"A kind gesture can reach a wound that only compassion can heal."*
>
> **STEVE MARABOLI**

Compassion is something this world has trouble understanding. The first reaction we often get when we are recommending Kangen Water® is suspicion. "Are you trying to sell me something?" people ask. It is hard for some to understand compassion. Willingness to help without any reward is weird to many. Very sad. Unless one helps without looking for a reward, one should just stay home and watch the box called TV. By looking at the box, one will stay in the box, however. Come out of the box!

There is a whole, beautiful world out there! People are sharing water like there is no tomorrow because they know what a difference it will make in people's lives.

Oh, and by the way, we do get paid by Enagic®. Let me remind you that so does your doctor, your pharmacist, your lawyer, every soda pop sales person, all the people who sell something weird and chewy (they call it macaroni and cheese), the vaccine pushers, and everyone else out there. Why shouldn't we get paid?

Why do Enagic® distributors get paid? Well, knowing a few hundred of them I would say because they are working hard, very hard at times, just like many others who educate, serve and have the guts to dream

The Purple Wave

about a better world. If you think that getting paid by Eangic® is easy money, why don't you join? See how 'easy' this type of work is. I am doing this work because I am passionate about it. I know quite a few other things would pay me more for less work but I chose Enagic® for many different reasons. Anyone can do the same. No resume, no university degree or special connection is needed. Some of us have higher education, simply because we were not born distributors. We all had to grow personally and professionally. We invested time in this and it was well worth it. If someone has a dream to do something beautiful, meaningful and make an honest living, this is the place to be. I firmly believe that Enagic®'s business model is the fairest and smartest way of allowing Kangen Water® users to share the exceptional quality and effectiveness of the products. Enagic® is an ethical and compassionate company. Everyone benefits in the greatest way. The water produced such profound results in people's lives that it's totally natural for them to share the benefits with their loved ones, friends and neighbors. They are simply rewarded financially because they care and they spread the word.

*"Where there is great love,
there are always miracles."*

WILLA CATHER

I feel privileged to be an ambassador for Enagic®. Making people aware and educating them about something this extraordinary is very fulfilling.

The 'Serenity Prayer' was on the wall in my bedroom for many years when I was so ill. I had to look at it every morning just to keep going. It goes like this: "God, grant me the serenity to accept the things I cannot change, courage to change the things I can and wisdom to know the difference."

I love the part 'courage to change the things I can'. I really embraced this in my life.

Friends, let's just change the things we can! Let's get into the forgotten habit of drinking good quality water. It is quite beautiful to live without a stroke. That might happen tomorrow or even tonight - not six months from now.

" I thrive in structure. I drown in chaos."

WATER

Just joking. This quote belongs to Anna Kendrick, but I am very suspicious that she heard this from water, as water would probably drown in its self without structure. LOL

If the genetic structure of the matter has changed so has its electrical structure and the body won't recognise it. It will reject it every time.

Some people think that science and miracles come from different places. There is only One Source! All that's true or worth looking at comes from *that* source. Yes, even miracles have to be reasonable. Are we?

"Miracles, do not in fact break the laws of nature."

C. S. LEWIS

CHAPTER 24

PEE AND POO EVERYWHERE!

"A long life may not be good enough, but a good life is long enough."

BENJAMIN FRANKLIN

Recently, special circumstances brought me to a place which looked like a luxury Hotel at first, with a reception, library, piano and even live music in the dining room but it turned out to be an 'assisted living' place or special accommodation for the elderly. I mostly saw men and women in wheelchairs or with walkers. We visited a woman who was only seven years older than me. My friend who was the same age as the woman, was hired to take care of this lady as she needed 'twenty-four-hour care'. It was difficult to watch what was happening. I will never forget the scene. A nurse came to medicate the woman. She did not want the pills. Another staff member came to ask about the next day's menu. She did not want anything from the menu. There was nothing natural or normal about the situation. The woman took off her diaper during the previous night and everything was soaking wet. The bed, the chairs in the living room, everything smelled like pee.

We saw the 'painted' walls. Guess what she used to paint the walls with? Her own poo! Yes, pee and poo were pretty much everywhere in the beautifully furnished apartment. I was stunned as I had never seen anything like this before.

I had to be 'educated' on the way of life of those people. They become so unreliable, crazy and weird that they need to be tied down and many of them won't recognise their life mates, their own caretaker or any of their family members. Heavy duty stuff. This is what we created. *This is what being on the wrong path in medicine looks like,* I am thinking. Those poor people are supposed to have all the wisdom of life and really enjoy the fruits of their labour at this time of life (their extra time, their grandchildren, their hard- earned money) and live or travel. Instead, they need twenty-four-hour care, which is exhausting and expensive for them and their relatives. This visit was a very sobering experience. I am hopeful that it won't happen to me. I know it won't happen. I have never taken a pain killer or a medication on a regular basis. I am looking forward towards my 'retirement' years. The best way to do retirement is by working a bit and having lots a healthy fun.

> *"First old woman: It's windy here.*
> *Second old woman: No, it's Thursday.*
> *Third old woman: I am thirsty too, let's have tea.*
> *First old woman: Oh good, I need to pee as well."*

UNKNOWN

It is funny and sad at the same time when old people can't hear each other and they still have an answer.

Besides hearing issues digestion problems can hit as well as we age. I used to think that digestion has everything to do with the food we eat. Now I know that good digestion depends on the water we are drinking and the pool of enzymes available in our body more so than the food we are eating. I believe that just as the seeds and nuts come to life when we soak them, this water does reactivate some of the enzymes in our body.

The Purple Wave

There is no other explanation for this. Before Kangen Water® I was unable to digest almost anything.

We learned from one of the biggest names in medicine, Dr. Hiromi Shinya, that enzymes are the source of life. This is true in plants and in people, as well. Dr. Shinya would not see a patient until they had been on a special diet drinking 'Kangen Water® for three months. Who are you listening to? We do not only kill the precious enzymes by over-cooking and processing the food we eat but we kill the enzymes in our body by not consuming water.

Now we can replace these marketed drinks, which have over the last 100 years replaced water. What a 'coincidence'! Only in the last 100 years have we been dealing with thousands of degenerative and especially neuro-degenerative problems.

To make the right choices, one needs some kind of clarity. Kangen Water® gave me much better clarity. One of the most painful things to see is young people being confused, suffering, stuck in wheelchairs, many with brain fog or migraines, depressed, drugged or hooked on alcohol, unable to learn and focus, addicted to pills or just vegetating. Life stops as soon as we stop learning and growing.

Using this ground-breaking technology, Enagic® succeeded in mimicking the Hunza water from nature. Exactly what Coanda wanted to re-create. He said: "Water contains within its structure the secret to reverse the aging process." Yes, it's not your plastic surgeon! It is Hydrogen, which is considered by the experts to be the missing link of longevity.

"Beautiful young people are accidents of nature, but beautiful old people are works of art."

ELEANOR ROOSEVELT

I have to tell you about the results from a new research, which involved the Germans and some international efforts, as well. A study by testing centenarians (people who live over 100 years) found only one common factor, which they all shared. Guess what it is? Not a good heart or liver, not exercise, diet or religion, not a nice family situation, not genetics, but 'Micro-Circulation'. We all have to have good circulation to live. Circulation, of course, involves water. Are you surprised? I am not. Not at all because I know what medical grade water, which significantly improves circulation in the body, can do. I also (finally) understand what lack of water does.

All the waters we have access to now, they all have a positive charge and an excess of H+ ions which makes the water acidic. The Hunza and Kangen Waters® are different. They have a negative charge and an excess of OH- ions, which gives the water a high pH. I had no idea about these things.

No wonder this type of water is happily accepted by our body. *"Molecular Hydrogen exhibits a very low ORP, and is thus a reducing agent or antioxidant. A low ORP is also seen with certain biological fluids, like the oral fluid of a healthy human and mother's milk for example, amniotic fluid, saliva, etc. as in the case of freshly made fruit or vegetable juice."* says Tyler LeBaron. Tyler W. LeBaron is the Founder and Executive Director of the science-based nonprofit Molecular Hydrogen Institute. His background is in biochemistry and exercise physiology. He speaks at Medical conferences in the US for doctors and at academic conferences around the world. He collaborates with researchers at home and abroad. He showed integrity in our conversations and as a scientist he is not endorsing any particular ionizer which is totally understandable. I heard this directly from his mouth.

What's left to do is to find out how you can get a reliable source of ionised water. You must be well-informed because it is an absolute Zoo out there when it comes to ionisers. People are really looking for ionised water. Some companies want to make quick money so they are trying hard to come up with different technology to imitate this water because the technology of the Kangen® machine is patented, of course (it cannot be copied). The only alternative they could come up with until this day is the so called 'mesh' technology and that turned out to be a disaster. You will learn why that is soon. It is not that easy to come up with new technology, which will produce the same outstanding result for less price. It is impossible to produce this machine for a lower price unless you compromise on the quality of the materials used. That is not recommended for obvious reasons.

Many are learning about this after the fact; after they've already spent a few thousand dollars on cheaper devices.

The Purple Wave

Some companies are changing the structure of the water to a degree but the water is still oxidising/acidic. Others are 'hydrogenising' the water but it is just as acidic as regular water and it has no negative charge. Most copycats are altering the water chemically to make it 'alkaline' but the water won't even absorb into the cells and has a positive charge. This is why it stays in your belly.

They all claim that they are as good as the 'gold standard' Enagic's famous SD 501. Even those who've never used our water have an opinion, so watch out...

> *"Smart people learn from everything and everyone. Average people from their experiences, stupid people already have all the answers."*
>
> **SOCRATES**

The philosopher Socrates lived long before political correctness came into style. Today stupid people don't want to be called stupid, which is understandable. Thankfully we don't have to stay stupid unless we want to be, of course. There is a free world our there. We can read, we can open our eyes, we can listen, we can turn the television off and we can trust Kangen Water®. Why?

Because The Japanese Association of Preventative Medicine for Adult Diseases fully endorses and approves it and have tested Enagic®'s Water Life Science Devices in clinical applications with their patients. This involved several thousands of doctors and hundreds of thousands of patients!

Even the plastic is medical grade! The strict standards and the Japanese precision have garnered awards and certificates, which are more than impressive and won't be found anywhere else.

I was truly impressed by this product when I first opened the box. More importantly, I am still impressed seven years later. I love to measure things by seeing how they stand the test of time. I've visited a few friends who bought other ionisers and learned that after a few months they were not happy. There was no negative charge, no hydrogen and more importantly there were no results.

One of the reasons why the Enagic® machines work continuously so well for many years is because they were built with conventional wisdom to last, paired with excellence of manufacturing practises and a simple but superior maintenance protocol.

Scam artists work overtime to convince you that there are cheaper or better ionisers on the market. No matter what the price is, those can't be taken apart and properly cleaned. As a consequence, they won't last. The so-called 'life-time warranty' is another scam. Every time a life time warranty is offered, you should run. Just think about it! Look and read the small print in the original warranty document. Always! You will realize that you can't find 'good enough' water, which will keep your warranty alive.

> ## "Strong brands are not built through shortcuts and copycats."
>
> **BERNARD KELVIN CLIVE**

Enagic® machines can be opened, taken into parts, which are individually replaceable and there is a serious but easy maintenance schedule you can follow to keep them free of calcium deposits and such. There are no moving parts inside. The after sales service is worth more than the actual price of the machine. This is just one of the reasons why you will need assistance after buying. Deal with someone who you have a relationship with and who is knowledgeable, who can train and educate you, test your water and help you with this new lifestyle.

Enagic® has no limitation on the water quality or the amount of water you can produce each day from the unit.

There are no hidden exclusions of anything in the contract or the warranty!

There are no surprises. You are dealing with the original equipment manufacturer and not a wholesaler changing their 'name' frequently hoping that they won't be found.

The Purple Wave

We never ask you to 'believe' anything, no empty promises; try the water yourself, experience it, enjoy it, play with it. Keep in touch with us. Contact Enagic®. We only ask you not to assume that the water from another ionizer is the same as the Kangen Water® you tried for three weeks. A common mistake people make. Other ionisers are sold instantly so people can't try the water. How convenient for the ioniser company. Not that great for the consumer.

Kangen Water® is produced solely by a Kangen® machine and they are made only by Enagic®.

Please visit our website to get a sense of the high ethics which govern this company and to see the prestigious certificates Enagic® has.

One is the totally unique Water Quality Association's Gold Seal Award for product certification as well as several International Standardization (ISO) Certificates. The website is well designed and easy to use but you really need a knowledgeable distributor with experience who is willing to guide you until you know how to get the most out of your machine. You will be provided with endless materials on the use of the different grades of waters. Get enlightened about all the technical data at www.enagic.com. You will be trained by your sponsor, how to do the proper maintenance, so your machine will keep producing the best water for decades. There is no middleman. Everything is backed by the manufacturer and it's easy to find them. Enagic® has service centers and well-trained technicians all around the globe. They can help you with information depending on your unique situation.

Are you getting closer in understanding why our water is the only one endorsed by the American Anti-Cancer Institute? All the different properties of the water work together to create amazing, some might say 'miraculous', results. Thankfully these properties can be measured so anyone can see how Kangen Water® measures, compared to everything else, with their own eyes. There are thousands of so called 'miracle' waters which will only lead to disappointment because they are not real. (natural) Of course there has to be a real one! That is the way nature intended water to be.

As we grow older our hydrogen pool becomes depleted and it is detrimental for the body. Our bodies get acidic; we can 'smell' this acidity in old age homes. This is that other smell I experienced besides the smell of pee and poo that day in this luxurious assisted living condominium.

It is well understood today that oxygen burns hydrogen in living systems, releasing much-needed energy for our bodies. So, to have energy, one needs hydrogen more than anything else. Again, no shortcuts in life.

> **"Yesterday's shortcuts are
> today's nightmares."**
>
> **MARK O'BRIEN**

CHAPTER 25

KILLER HABITS

"We are what we repeatedly do.
Excellence then, is not an act, but a habit."

ARISTOTLE

Ever since I was a child, I always wanted to excel in everything I did. I remember that I was encouraged by my parents, but it was more than that. I was ambitious, I did work hard and I was first in my class in grade one, then second in grade two, third in grade three. As I was growing up, things changed a little bit in that regard. I could never achieve 100 percent excellence after age 12. I became weaker in all my performances. In high school I dropped to fifth or sixth place. At college I was near the bottom. Something was hindering me. It felt that my own mind was stopping me from being 'the best' or better than I was. Today, so many years later, as weird as it sounds, I know that yes, indeed it was my brain, my dehydrated brain. I discovered something interesting as I looked into dehydration and listened to many experts. The reason my mind did not let me 'go all the way' and I was performing less and less, making not so great decisions at times, was the result of gradual cumulative dehydration. This ended up causing more serious problems in my twenties and my thirties. I am certain about this now.

The habit of not drinking enough water after age twelve when I got very ill from bad quality water interfered with my life in unpredictable ways. Over the course of our lives we develop (for many different reasons) habits that do not serve us well. Just the opposite: they become obstacles in achieving our goals and dreams.

What can we do when we become captives of bad habits? Often in life we point to others, we turn somewhere else for direction but the truth is that the person responsible and the one who can do something about it, is the 'person in the mirror.'

Where to start? There are many opinions on this subject. First, of course, we have to have faith that we can do the task to change our habits... once we are conscious about them. That is pretty much the same with everything we do. Why would bad habits be any different?

**"Believe you can and you're
halfway there."**

THEODORE ROOSEVELT

Okay, I take that. 50 percent is good enough to start. Only 50 percent left and that is a 'piece of cake'. As soon as I believed that I can drink this water, I was drinking it.

**"The first step towards getting
somewhere is to decide that you
are not going to stay where you are."**

UNKNOWN

The place where I found myself at age 57 was a very scary one. I thought for a while that my life as I knew it was really over. *Yes, but this early in life?* I was thinking. *Wow, I will be very soon this old 'babushka' with canes, caretakers and diapers with millions of wrinkles on my face*

The Purple Wave

and who knows what else. One thing, which really scared me was that I had a very hard time holding my urine.

I had a very bad habit and I never though about it. I forgot all about drinking water. I hated water.

> *"Bad habits are spiraling slides that drag you round and round down the narrowing end of a cone that eventually ends up in a dark, tight, confining spot... Bad habits are demons that often push us into isolation because they know that in our loneliness they stand little chance of being overcome."*

> RICHELLE E. GOODRICH

From everything we 'modern' humans routinely do, to knowingly or unknowingly destroy or abuse ourselves, which is considered a wrong attitude or a bad habit, the worst by far is (that includes smoking) the horrible habit of not drinking enough water.

By avoiding water for forty-five years, I did find myself in isolation. No one knew about what was happening to me including myself. My first hospitalization happened around age seventeen when 'I couldn't breathe'. My Mom took me to a few doctors with no results. No cause was found. I stayed two weeks under the supervision of an old doctor in Tirgu Mures. The city was famous for having the best hospitals. He came up with a diagnosis, quite close to the truth: "Calcium deficiency", which of course would not happen if I was drinking enough water. For a few years I was given the calcium intravenously. Dehydration or water was never mentioned. For forty-five years I did not find water that I liked or could drink except carbonated bottled mineral water when I felt thirst.

> *"Good habits are hooked wings, that steadily grow in girth and strength. At first, they grasp and climb until those beautiful wings can lift*

Klara Reid

the bearer out of the darkness and above the clouds to heights few ever experience."

RICHELLE E. GOODRICH

Forty-five years later when I started to drink this superior quality water, I instantly enjoyed it. I had no problem drinking it. It was surprisingly smooth and light. Not long after that I started to see the results and the benefits were definitely worth the effort. Until this day, I love this water. I was blessed by this change of a habit, 'tenfold'.

"The secret to permanently breaking any bad habit is to love something greater than the habit."

BRYANT MCGILL

I had to reconsider my relationship with water.

I love the way I feel and perform now. I travel with my machine and I am always well hydrated. This new habit and the amazing water saved me from lots of headaches, injuries, blood clots, brain fog, flu, inflammation, you name it. With the different grades of water, I take care of infections, bites, burn, fungus, contagious conditions, pesticides, heavy metal poisoning and much more.

'The purple wave' lifted me by giving me 'the wings' I needed to get into the forgotten habit of drinking water again.

Finally, I got my life back! I am experiencing the amazing feeling of *"flying above the clouds, to heights few ever experience"*. Kangen Water® is something I will never give up voluntarily. That is exactly what you might be missing, my friend. You also have it in you to change your habits. You got this far by reading the book, right? Make sure that your time wasn't wasted.

> *"Most people don't have that willingness to break bad habits. They have a lot of excuses and they talk like victims."*
>
> **CARLOS SANTANA**

Yes, the majority do have excuses but you are not a victim. We agreed earlier that you shouldn't be part of the majority. You got help from above. I bet you did more outrageous things, tried riskier adventures than water drinking.

Kangen Water® was a game changer for us as a family, as Fred, my husband says!

Kangen Water® is by far the best solution for addictions, I have seen so far!

Switching from two liters of soda (that was *his* bad habit) to three liters of Kangen Water® made a world of difference in his life. The same is true with other addictions like sugar, food, cigarettes, alcohol or coffee. This water makes the replacement of these with water so much easier.

Don't say or think anything until you actually try it! You won't get bloated, it won't fill you with plastic, or chlorine. It won't deprive you from your mineral reserves, it will nourish your craving body better than anything else.

It might be the time for you to do a 'self-evaluation'. We all have to do that from time to time. We have to change our mindset, renew our minds. Some call bad habits a 'sin'. I don't. God-loving, self respecting, intelligent people know that they were born to be victorious, not victims. Bad habits are as the name says, only habits. Habits can be changed. Sometimes, it's not easy, still many quit smoking, for example.

Addictions are hard to get rid of. New habits, however can be easily implemented. We just have to get off 'autopilot', evaluate our routines or the behavior we are used to and adjust ourselves. I needed to change my drinking habit big time. I would never have realised how dehydrated I was and what all my problems were rooted in if I did not go to a Kangen® event. So, if you never have seen one, please do yourself a favor and go as soon as possible. If no one invited you yet, I will invite you. We can do a webinar together or something of that sort. Go before the stroke or the insulin. Go for yourself and not for the person who is inviting you.

" You cannot change your future, but you can change your habits, and surely your habits will change your future."

DR. ABDUL KALAM

Let's say an 'amen' to that.

CHAPTER 26

CRAZY OR THIRSTY CHILDREN?

"They are much to be pitied who have not been given a taste for nature in life."

JANE AUSTEN

The taste of water might not be part of the "taste of nature" for the generations to come if we continue this nonsense. It makes my blood boil when I see what most of the children are drinking today. Everyone makes money on these and that's what really matters, I think. Every store, every restaurant, every vending machine, airports, hospitals, everything is filled with plastic bottles. When I was growing up, these were non-existent and we managed. Imagine how 'cheap' this stuff initially is. The profit margins must be huge. They don't have to 'manufacture' the water, they just fill up millions of bottles every day destroying the vital water sources of locals in the most irresponsible way. To manufacture each bottle, however, a quarter bottle of petroleum is used. No comment! Insanity goes far these days. I seen bottled water sold in stores in BC, the land of amazing source water, from Quebec, which is 6000 km's away.

Childhood is when parents should focus and assist children in 'building' a strong immune system by giving the child the best of nutrition and of course love and attention. We see so many ill children today. We see kids in wheelchairs, bald from chemo, not able to perform in school. We see children who are constipated [I know this as I was one of them growing up. Always constipated and I never told anyone until I got married.] who are 'treated' with pills instead of water! The parents don't know better, the school doesn't know better and the health-care providers don't know better. What to do in this absurd situation?

*"Education should be Exercise;
it has become 'massage'."*

MARTIN H. FISCHER

Today's kids are out of control because they **don't drink water!** Their brain is starving and they drive parents and teachers crazy. Their diet is full of junk and on top of that there is no flushing, detoxing and no hydration. How can they be healthy or function properly, I ask?

I don't really understand this part of the deal. I see horrible neglect and ignorance with some parents. My main concern is that the next generation does not have much choice. If these precious children are being offered only sugary and acidic drinks, junk to eat they have no chance. My heart is bleeding. Kids today have many 'things', much more than what we or our kids had. They are spoiled with clothing, cell phones and other stuff, games, electronics, things they might want but don't necessarily need.

They need water! They need good quality water.

Water, nutrition, love, discipline and education in that order! Parents are not getting much help from the school or the governments. Schools became dangerous. From bullying to shootings from liberal ideas to lack of respect and discipline, everything goes. What can we expect?

The Purple Wave

> *"There can be no keener revelation*
> *of a society's soul than the way in*
> *which it treats its children"*
>
> **N. MANDELA**

I am worried about young athletes, dancers and teenagers in general. Often these athletes are practically destroyed by the sport drinks they ingest, which dehydrate them to the point of having concussions. They lose so much water that the 'cushioning' around the brain (cerebrospinal fluids) becomes so thin it doesn't protect the brain from physical trauma, which they have a lot of. In this crazy competitive world, most sports have lost their initial purpose. I imagine that people do sports to have physical fitness, not to become disabled before they turn thirty. Huge individual lawsuits and class actions are happening one after the other. The 'law' never goes after those responsible! Everyone is blamed except those who are behind these aggressive corporations. The problem never gets solved as no one is addressing the root causes.

At times we hear that children drop dead as the 'energy' drinks are becoming stronger and more addictive. A preventable problem but only for those who have the proper knowledge, wisdom and care.

> *"Children must be taught how to*
> *think, not what to think."*
>
> **MARGARET MEAD**

Water should be the number one nutrient for your kids, as well. The number one nutrient! This means that your kids should drink enough water and quality water, which will do the job. Your kids should stay away from sodas and marketed garbage. It doesn't matter what colour or what the name is' if it comes in a plastic bottle, it's poison. To achieve this it's hard, of course, almost impossible, unless you have something to replace it with.

The only reason I was successful in getting some of my family members to drop marketed drinks was because of Kangen Water®.

Both my husband and daughter replaced all the sodas with Kangen Water®. It was simple enough. Our grandkids love the water. This doesn't mean that we are not drinking occasionally a beer or a glass of wine, a fruit juice or something, but we will never replace water.

We are having an 'unseen epidemic' when it comes to society at large. It is not contagious, but the behaviour or the 'lifestyle' that causes the tragedy of collective bad health is indeed contagious.

Kids imitate big sport stars and celebrities who shamelessly advertise these drinks because they get paid big money.

The parents are not educated or they don't have much influence in the family. Sad, sad situation. Your child doesn't have to become a victim, now that you found out about this. They might not listen to you but you can do what I did with my adult children. I asked them nicely to go and get informed, in fact I made it mandatory for them. I told them after they get informed, they can choose whatever they think is best for them. They did not like the idea and they dumped the 'no time' BS on me but I was firm. They went, they tried the water and they loved it. Simple. So, dehydration is ancient history in my family and I am very grateful for that.

We must do everything in our power to stop the insanity.

Imagine this: only two percent drop in water intake will result in a twenty percent reduction of mental and physical performance. Do you know why your kid has challenges, is depressed or underperforming in school? You might want to check his/her natural water intake and everything else he/she is drinking.

Many kids are addicted to these drinks. It is an absolute nightmare when this happens as these products cause everything from cancer to diabetes, obesity and more. It is easy to get addicted to them. The best and fastest way (in my humble opinion, the only way) to get rid of this addiction is: **to offer an alternative! They can't just stop drinking. They have to replace it with something better!**

This worked well when I got the machine, way above my expectations. In a matter of two or three weeks, both my daughter and my husband forgot all about sodas. This could have not been done with anything else! I know it. We tried it many times before.

There is something else most families don't suspect or talk about. The poisonous chemicals sprayed on everything - the fruits, the nuts, the veggies. When my kids were babies, in the early 80s, I was told by our pediatrician that I must safeguard them so they are not poisoned by the chemicals used in agriculture. She was dead serious, she demanded I remove the skin off the tomatoes for example. We strictly followed her instructions. Kids are extremely vulnerable as their immune system is not fully developed. Their bodies don't know how to fight these poisons.

Dr. IRENKE, (we called her by her first name) expressed her concern about what is coming in terms of world contamination. She was (we thought at the time) 'paranoid' about these chemicals. Spraying started in the 70s in Romania if I remember correctly, exactly when our kids were born. My parents did not have to deal with this issue when we were kids. We needed education.

"Liberal use of pesticides in food crops is a major threat to brain health. Children are particularly vulnerable to the brain damaging effects of toxic pesticides."

DR. LYON

In his book called "Is Your Child's Brain Starving?" Dr. Michael R. Lyon, a medical researcher states: "It will take years, maybe even decades, for these harmful agents to be eliminated from our food supply." His book was published in 2002. Seventeen years after his book was published, the food producers are using not less but more and more of these poisons, as you can very well see. Much more! It seems that this 'organised crime' won't stop anytime soon. Accurate statistics from the USA:

"In 2006 and 2007, 1.5 billion pounds of pesticides were used".

Imagine that. It is insane to intentionally destroy the environment and people's lives. Look what is happening today! Chemicals and cell phones are killing our children.

Cancer is the number one killer of children under age fourteen. Now you know where cancer is coming from.

It is hard for some to comprehend that everything goes through us, everything found in our environment, everything.

When I was so ill that I almost died from mercury and other poisonous metals, the bio-dentist who removed the amalgam from my mouth gave me a warning. "Stay away from pesticides if you want to live. They are made of heavy metals you don't want more of in your system." I will never forget this warning. I purchased the Kangen® machine so we can eat pesticides free food.

Since 2012, I have faithfully used the 11.5 pH water from my Kangen® machine to remove all the toxic chemicals from the food we eat and it has made a world of difference. I love my family. It only takes an extra five to ten minutes a day to prepare clean food for our table.

I sincerely hope and pray that parents will smarten up quickly or there will be no next generation!

Water is the one universal component that is essential for both the mental and physical strength of children!

The Kangen® machine is the only reasonable and affordable tool to provide pesticide free food for the family.

"It is easier to build strong children
than to repair broken man."

FREDERICK DOUGLASS

CHAPTER 27

BUSINESS AS USUAL, OR SOMETHING EXTRAORDINARY?

*"Think of energy almost like emotional electricity.
It has a powerful way of uniting ordinary people,
their connected spirit, to do extraordinary things."*

ANGELA AHRENDTS

Through Enagic® we met and connected with 'ordinary people' who are doing truly extraordinary things. *We are* now doing things, which are 'extraordinary'.

I talked about love and water separately. Let's unite the two. So, you are getting a gallon of this water handed to you with love. Why is this important? You can see how water reacts to feelings, emotions, music and such by looking at the famous water crystal photos, the work of Dr. Masaru Emoto (1943-2014). His degree was from the University of Yokohama, Japan. He was considered a pseudoscientist who proved by photos (never good enough for some of the scientific community) that human consciousness has an effect on the molecular structure of water.

Emoto's book "*The Hidden Messages in Water*" was a New York Times best seller.

When we give away water with love and compassion, as our C.E.O., Mr. Ohshiro intended, that water has everything! It will react to our 'frequency' or 'emotional electricity' and it will have what we have in our hearts. Intention matters and it matters a lot. I know that. That gallon of water already has the power to help the body to heal because it has the purity, the right structure, it has the negative charge, it has the minerals we need and it has the Hydrogen. It will do its job. Now, when you pray over it, you intend love and compassion, it will have the right sparks, the 'right attitude', as well. This is already the 'spiritual realm'. Please don't forget about the 'why' or the reason you are giving out water. It is to make someone better and to make them happy. Two universal things, love and water beautifully assembled together. I am not a painter but I know that on a canvas, this combination would be one amazing picture. No wonder we feel like we are on top of the world when we are drinking this water and giving it away freely with love and compassion.

This happened to me. Someone, a stranger at the time, but a friend ever since and forever (Sabine Gaudette) handed my husband a gallon of water and that changed everything. I will never forget that. I will be grateful to her forever. She shared this water because she'd seen the amazing results her husband was having by drinking it. I felt that love.

Love is truly extraordinary, it transcends, we usually say. It will 'transfigure', for lack of a better word, from physical to spiritual or vice versa. It might just be that water is the 'medium' through which this is possible. Wow! Are you still ignoring water? All we aim to do is help people who need help, who are looking for help or who would accept help! Love should be above all things and this is the way it was with Sabine. I hope that love is felt and recognized when I am recommending this water.

From the business perspective, it might be that lack of love is why some people aren't successful. They consider selling Kangen machines a 'job'.

I just don't want people to suffer unnecessarily! There are plenty of other problems. This is my 'Why.'

This is why every morning, as soon as I get up, I ask this simple question: Who might benefit from our water? It is up to the person if

The Purple Wave

she/he believes me or not but I feel that sharing this water and this mind-blowing information with others is a gift for them. The results I see are 'recharging' me day after day. I was blessed with mentors in the business who were and are caring people. They understood from the beginning that this is about changing lives. There is a reason why the company is simply asking you to "Change your water," as we know that it will "Change your life".

Now, imagine this: You have a situation where you've finally found something unique, phenomenal, long-lasting, of the highest quality and universal. 99 percent of the population desperately needs it. It's not just another product.

You are addressing a tremendous need. You are solving serious problems for people.

"Take advantage of big trends ... look below the surface ... that is where you can find Big Ideas. There are demographics, cultural, financial, technological and medical trends in place now that will produce predictable results years from now."

DONALD J. TRUMP

I truly believe that this was written by a 'business genius', of course.

There are huge opportunities when it comes to intellectual distribution. Today 53 percent of businesses are home based. Are you aware of the opportunity Enagic® represents? My husband and I considered selling the Enagic® products only after using it for over a year. This wasn't planned, at all. We saw the results and those prompted us to share it with others. It turned out to be a viable business opportunity for our retirement. We are successful and we are selling globally now. You can contact us from any country. We are part of this 'big solution' for an accelerated human need. It feels good. You too can take advantage of this cultural shift. It only has just begun. People are thinking more ecologically now; we have some smart and environmentally sound young people as well, not only brain washed ones. 'Paradigm shift' means "Change in people's perception and people's ideas. A time when the usual and accepted way of doing and thinking about something changes completely". It is quite well defined by the encyclopedia. This new way of thinking will bring physical, economical and other changes.

Enagic® has had no real competition for over forty years now and chances are, we won't have any for a long time. Market penetration is only half a percent in some areas and generally between 1-2 percent globally. If you can imagine this situation, you will realise that this is a once in a life time opportunity and your work will be fulfilling and appreciated. Now you can understand why I am excited. I am not going to run out of work and excitement any time soon.

> *"We each have a special something we can get only at a special time of our life. Like a small flame. A careful, fortunate few cherish that flame, nurture it, hold it as a torch to light their way."*
>
> **HARUKI MURAKAMI**

This beautiful quote might express how special and important this new 'way of life' is for me.

I recently spent two days at the Canadian National Pickle Ball Tournament in Kelowna, BC. I was very surprised how many people had 'energy drinks', sodas and plastic water in their hands. We are talking about the baby boomer generation; they should know better! They need the boost of electrolytes to have energy for playing but they have no idea what harm these beverages cause. Many of them had knee and ankle bandages, wrist bandages, arthritis pain, artificial knees and hips, osteoporosis and none of them suspect what is the main contributing factor to their problems. They are constantly losing precious minerals from their bones and muscles. Many of them are on pills. They are nice, fun loving people who understand the need of exercise. They however overlook hydration or have no idea how to get hydrated. They get injured one after the other and it takes them forever to heal.

The sciatic nerve will cause horrible pain when a person gets dehydrated as the 'cushioning' around the nerves disappears. I used to have sciatic pain. Not anymore.

The Purple Wave

Injury is not fun, especially if the body doesn't have the surplus energy to heal. I find it sad that some people fear knowledge more than they fear cancer or injury. There is a documentary called: "Escape Fire; The fight to Rescue American Healthcare." It is mind-blowing how many people die from infections and medical errors or interventions they don't really need.

I am so blessed. Would you believe me if I told you that I live with permanent heart damage? This condition I have for fifteen years now is called "left anterior hemi block", a fairly serious problem, which was more than scary before I began drinking Kangen Water®. Dehydration during chelation was the cause, I think. I did not even know at the time that I have to drink tons of water and the Naturopath doctor who did a 'new method' of chelation did not tell me either, nor did I have Kangen Water®. Anyhow, my heart was damaged as a result. This condition means a failure of 'cardiac impulses.' The heart has electrical circuitry and in the case of a hemi block, there is a short circuit in the heart created by a heart attack, which happens during sleep or something of that sort. The symptoms are very scary. For about six years, at many times, I was running to the emergency of different hospitals in the middle of the night. All that is history now. Since I began drinking electrolysed water, I am no longer on supplement pills or co-enzyme Q10. I seldom need to take calcium/magnesium anymore. I could not exist without spending about $250/month on Q10, Calcium, Magnesium and other expensive supplements. I have a normal life as somehow my heart has enough energy and works, thanks to the water. Magnesium used to help me, however, I also had to come up with that solution myself as the heart specialist "wasn't allowed to comment" on any of my questions regarding supplementation. I can't explain to you what is happening with my heart muscle. I am a simple user of the water, not a doctor, remember? I can truthfully say, however, that it feels like I have a normal heart as my heart is not 'misbehaving' as long as I drink my water.

This is what I call a Miracle. I might be the only person with this condition who is living a normal life without a pace maker. This idea of electrolyzed water for people with a faulty electrical conduction in the heart is something which just fell into my lap. I only had to recognize it and I did. I took a chance and it worked, besides, you can't go wrong with good water.

Klara Reid

I don't know, of course, for how long my heart will keep 'pumping' to keep me alive but I am grateful that it did work until now so I could tell my story.

> **"When 99% of people doubt your idea, You're either gravely wrong or about to make history."**
>
> *SCOTT BELSKY*

I am also grateful for leading research and researchers who are discovering these biologically significant applications of the water molecule. I am very grateful to all the airport security personnel who let me bring plenty of my water on board after testing it as I travel by air frequently. I wish all travelers would have access to this water on board, especially the pilots. Perhaps many strokes, blood clots, or even tragic disasters in aviation could be avoided. I am sure that is coming. After all, NASA astronauts are risking their own lives only when they fly and they are drinking structured water for months before they take off to space. Why not pilots who are risking millions of lives? **Attention Airlines!**

Kangen Water® came into my life at the right moment when I could not endure arthritis pain any longer. I also have gout and at times I experience mild pain when I don't drink enough water. This is my reminder to drink more. After eight months of drinking three to four liters per day of Kangen Water®, the arthritis pain ceased completely. I never expected this but it did happen**. I call this an absolute blessing.** Many were prompted to put their testimonials up on YouTube. I did not. I just wrote my story for others to read.

According to Dr. Hidemitsu Hayashi, Director of the Water Institute of Japan, *"We must work on the problems upstream at the headwaters -the source of pollution - not downstream where we can only try to treat the evidence of damage caused by the pollution. Ionized water's contribution to preventative medicine is essentially an upstream treatment."* The Japanese say: "We consider the digestive track upstream, where we intake water and food. Many people today tend to concentrate more on what the food contains, rather than the metabolised products of foods in the digestive tract."

I think this is the answer many are looking for.

The Purple Wave

Some of us, of course, have an Enagic® machine, but we are not nearly enough in numbers to make an impact on the environment, which is one of our ultimate goals. This is where the opportunity for you lies.

Martin Luther King Jr. said "The ultimate measure of a man is not where he stands in moments of comfort, but where he stands at times of challenge and controversy." Where do you stand?

Let me know if you want to join the movement.

I will talk about this for the rest of my life. I experienced a waterborne illness, which almost killed me. I went through the dry years and countless hospitalizations. Then, I experienced how water can help the body by assisting the immune system. There is no better way to express how grateful I am for my health.

**"In our woundedness, we can
become sources of life for others."**

HENRY J NOUVEN

There are many good people on this Earth and now you can see that there is good water, as well.

Being passionate is considered weird by some. It is the official 'diagnosis' people put on me but I don't put it on myself. To me, sharing the truth is natural. It can be anything, not necessarily water. Yes, I might sound crazy at times but there are worse things than that. One would be to look 'normal'. Oh, that sounds awfully boring. LOL.

**"The ones who are crazy enough to
think that they can change the
world, are the ones who do."**

STEVE JOBS

I am open to people and I'm open to new ideas.

This is what I call Life. I would like to mention here, that Kangen water® doesn't cure anyone nor did it cure me. I still have a weakened immune system from all what happened to me. I will never be cured. I understand that. I however can manage my health well without drugs and I don't have to deal with the side effects later. My body never accepted dead water from a plastic bottle or tap water.

Many are offended when they find out that their health can't be taken for granted and that they must invest greatly in their own and their family's health. Everyone is looking for money! My father used to say "As long as I am healthy, I am rich."

Money will only be worth less and less in the future. Water, good food, time off work, will be worth more and more. So, why not look for health instead of money?

I meet so many people who are 'planning' to get healthy, planning to find a healthier source for their water, planning to change their habits, to eat right, to become a better person. They get the theory part but they absolutely don't understand how to take action, now!

> *"A lot of people have ideas, but there are few who decide to do something about them, now! Not tomorrow, not next week, but TODAY!"*
>
> **NOLAN BUSHNELL**

With these experiences - which I have shared with you - I have learned how water can kill, how water can help heal, or how lack of water can make one's life hardly livable.

Nothing is as expensive as a missed opportunity. If I had focused on my 'assets', our house, the new SUV we had just purchased and everything else that was going on in my life, I am certain I would have missed a tremendous opportunity life presented to me at the right time. I was approaching 60 and instead of the 'stuff' I embraced the water. I never looked back. I love everything that came with it; the company, the people we have attracted, this honest and hard work, the learning and everything else, even the difficulties. It felt good to struggle for a while.

The Purple Wave

We surrounded ourselves with real people who we could count on, people who lifted us up, helped us grow and prosper. Prosperity is more than money, you see. Real 'prosperity' is finding your place in life, feeling great on this Earth and in the business world. It felt amazing when we overcame the obstacles. I was getting better and better from the water and we became happier and happier, quite often thrilled by seeing others having results. Our relationship also got strengthened. The water came not long after Fred and I met and got married so it was the beginning of a new life on more than one level. Everything we did, we did it together. We supported each other. We grew together, we cheered together. At times we 'went crazy' together as we struggled financially. We travelled together. We got repeatedly separated as I started traveling across the country to spread the news and plant seeds. One day we just realised that we are living the very life we first talked about, we just had no idea how to get there. That just happened automatically. This water brought us where we wanted to go, exactly where we wanted to be. Thank you Enagic®. Thanks for being more, much more than a business. Thank you for being something 'extraordinary'!

What is extraordinary? Working for a company which is all about making money is ordinary. Not being your own boss is ordinary. Being stuck in traffic almost every day is ordinary. We are done with ordinary, 'we arrived', thanks to Kangen Water® and I find this completely, totally and absolutely (as Fred likes to say) extraordinary.

"The past cannot be changed.
The future is yet in your power!"

UNKNOWN

CHAPTER 28

PRICE OR VALUE?

*"Price is what you pay, and
value is what you get."*

WARREN BUFFETT

Warren Buffett should be believed when it comes to money. He needs no 'introduction' that's how rich he is, so don't expect one. The price and the value of something usually match but sometimes, we pay a higher price for certain things than what they are worth. I am thinking about a car. When you buy it new, the price is quite high. As soon as it's driven out of the dealership, the value drops sometimes by over $10,000. People still buy new cars, of course. Let's see how much a smart phone or smart communication cost today? Fred and I will pay $72,000 to Bell in the next thirty years. Every month we are charged $100.00 CAD, for our smart phones each of us separately. That is the price. I am not sure about the value we are getting for it. What do you think?

As Mr. Buffet says: "The price is what we pay, the value is what we are getting." In the case of a Kangen® machine, things are very different. Its value is much higher than its price in my humble opinion. Much higher. I know the value of this medical device from my own experience.

The Purple Wave

How about the price of the Kangen®machine, compared to another ioniser? Oh, this is a no brainer. I am sure you know basic math? If you do, you will never buy into ordinary ionisers. Which is more? Spending $4,000 once in twenty-five years (that is the lifespan of the Kangen® machine) or $2,600 every two years? (that's the average time ordinary ionisers are used) Do the math! Why aren't these ionisers used after a year or two? Very simple. No ORP or negative charge, no H2, no excitement. They are forgotten even if they don't break but most of them do or the unit becomes soggy and moldy as they can't be cleaned. They are forgettable. For that short of a lifespan, and no significant results, I consider ordinary ionisers extremely expensive but that is just me. I work hard for my money. Kangen® machines on the other hand are unforgettable. More than that, they are irreplaceable, once we use them.

But is it price you should be concerned about when your life or wellbeing is at stake? How much is your life worth? It is silly to talk about price when it comes to health, of course. Human life is priceless. Human life is also fragile. It can be over in a matter of seconds.

The value of the Kangen® machine is this; not having one can and will cost hundreds, or thousands of dollars in health-related bills, time lost from work, meds, wheelchairs, sleep apnea machines, surgeries, disability and other expenses. Life will just cost more from day to day and everyday, if you have to purchase all the things you can easily replace by the waters.

This is precisely the value of it and it is the main reason why over 1.5 million people already have purchased it.

It is the best investment by far anyone can make at any time!

*"Good health is not something we can buy.
However, it can be an extremely
valuable savings account."*

ANNE WILSON SCHAEF

In her amazing Journal called, "Conquering Stroke", Valerie Greene, whose recovery surpassed even the most optimistic expectations, shares her testimony of how water helped her. Kangen Water® was her number one choice to obtain maximum brain function again, after a stroke.

I personally know a few other people whose recovery after strokes have been remarkable. What we are seeing, what is marvellous, is that stroke patients who regularly drink the water might just prevent future strokes. That is huge because usually strokes are followed by more strokes. I personally think that it is good to buy the machine before the first stroke, not after, but that is just me. I love to be able to move around and have a full life.

Now you know the value of the ultimate 'health machine'.

Now, it is okay to ask me about the price. Soon you understand the value, you will clearly see how ridiculously low the price is.

Imagine finding out that a car will cost $38,000 before you find out what it can do for you! I am sure you would run out of the dealership if the car appeared to you as four chairs assembled together, not knowing that it can move and take you places. In the same way, some people just run when they hear about the price of this medical device, knowing nothing about what it can do for their family.

This is doing things backwards, I think.

Instead of looking into a different idea, some are buying 'smart' water. It might cost them three dollars for the bottle. I would like them to know, with all due respect, that the water is not working for them. I mean they are not getting any 'smarter' from it! I just love simple and practical things.

How much money do you think you can save in a few years using this new tool? It depends how much money you are spending right now on drugs and supplements that aren't really helping you. My husband Fred and I have saved a minimum of $500.00 CAD every month since we have the device in the kitchen. We no longer spend on different drugs, enzymes, supplements, or on products like rubbing alcohol, window cleaner, air freshener, make-up remover, mouthwash and so on. This doesn't include the thousands we've saved by not going to a veterinary clinic with our dog for five years.

"People do not buy goods and
services. They buy relations,
stories and magic."

SETH GODIN

The Purple Wave

Oh, this never been more true than in the case of buying a Kangen machine.

Dr. Mu Shik Jhon has devoted his life to assembling the pieces of "The Water Puzzle" together. He tells us that what makes vitamin C so powerful is that it changes the structure of pentagonal water into hexagonal water. Wow. Thank you, Mu Shik Jhon, for your tremendous contribution. I am not sure if he and his discovery are appreciated enough!

This is why drinking Hexagonal or Structured water is so important.

It makes sense. Isn't the Creator who created both the human body and the ultimate fuel for us truly a genius? How dare some think that they can do better. **I call that an *insult* to the maker.**

Water is called the 'blue gold' but, of course, it's much more valuable than gold. Some closed-minded people are still in the dark causing confusion about water in this otherwise enlightened era!

Dr. Batmanghelidj, the 'water doctor', has saved 3,000 inmates' lives in an Iranian jail with water only! He was genuine and a real researcher, besides being an M.D. Fereydoon Batmanghelidj was born in Iran, in 1931. He practiced medicine in the United Kingdom. Dr. Batmanghelidj discovered the healing powers of water when he was serving as a political prisoner in jail. He stayed an additional six months as a volunteer after he was let go, so he could finish his research. Several months later he came to America to further research and eventually introduce his medical discovery to scientists and researchers in the United States. The report about his findings was published in the "Journal of Clinical Gastroenterology", in June of 1983. Amazing story. The 'New York Times' Science Watch also reported this discovery on June 21st of the same year. He is called "crazy and irresponsible" by some but I trust him. The crazier, the better, I think. LOL. At the Foundation for the Simple in Medicine, he began to research the effect of chronic unintentional dehydration on the human body. His ground breaking work was published again, this time, in the Foundation's "Journal of Science in Medicine Simplified," in 1991 and 1992.

I went through most of the conditions he is talking about in his book (pain, arthritis pain, dyspeptic pain, hiatus hernia, false appendicitis pain, anginal pain, asthma, allergies, overeating, panic attacks, to name a few) so I have the ultimate proof that he is indeed a genius.

Let's see another perspective, from a totally different source.

We learned from Dr. Filtzer that the mitochondria (the cell engines) are helped by Kangen Water® in measurable and significant ways.

Klara Reid

Tory Hagen, a researcher at the Linus Pauling Institute in Corvallis, Oregon who probably doesn't even know about Kangen Water® says: "The mitochondria has been called the Achilles heel of the cells in aging. Precious things come in small packages, and there's no better example than mitochondria. Each cell in our body contains up to 2,000 mitochondria and, although tiny, they make up to 60 percent of the volume of muscle cells and forty percent of heart cells." This is true agelessness.

Now I kind of understand why my weak (damaged by mercury) heart is helped so much by Kangen Water®. Wow. The 'turbines' in my heart are powered by this water.

Mr. Melov, Director of the Genomics Core at the Buck Institute for Age Research, reports, "Mitochondria are the power plants of our cells, tiny furnaces within the cells of our body that burn food for energy."

To do this, I suppose you need water. Lots of functional water.

Do you see the connection? Hydrogen is called longevity's missing link for a reason. The good news is that you already know about it. At one point in my life when I needed this more than anything else, I was blessed by this water. Things, which seemed complicated, (a handful of auto-immune problems I had) got solved because of curiosity about something simple enough. I hope I made your decision easier for you. I love revelations, all the 'help' coming from within and I love natural solutions because they can't hurt. I want to help everyone. Do you think that is weird?

> *"To solve a difficult problem in medicine,*
> *don't study it directly, but rather pursue*
> *a curiosity about nature and*
> *the rest will follow."*
>
> **ROGER KORNBERG Ph.D.**
> **Stanford School of Medicine**

Wow. Seriously? Looks like I am not that weird after all. I did just that. This is unbelievable but it is true. My personal search for natural solutions did lead to the answer. I had no idea about this 'idea' of Dr. Kornberg's,

The Purple Wave

I have just found this quote. I instinctively followed the same idea seven years ago. Because of my curiosity in the science of water, "the rest did follow". I kind of feel very special right now. The truth, however, is that it's not me. I mean I am 'special' but not that special. It was all God, nature, water, and compassionate people. I know that even wisdom and faith is coming from God. I can't take credit for any of these.

CHAPTER 29

YOUR HEART AND THE MEDIA

*"Manipulating the media is akin to poisoning
a nation's water supply. It affects all
of our lives in unimaginable ways."*

LANCE MORCAN

No kidding! When we know that the number one killer is heart disease, heart attacks, heart failure and such, we should seek at least *some* understanding of the causes.

In this chapter, we will see that oxidation and dehydration as mentioned before are the root causes of heart attacks. Yes, not stress, not cholesterol, not fat, or anything like that. The truth is, that the body starts making cholesterol in order to protect the artery walls from dehydration and oxidation. The heart is the most alkalinity-dependent of all organs.

You are scammed and doomed at the same time if you are taking (super acidic) prescription pills permanently after a heart episode and you will pay dearly for that decision!

The Purple Wave

This should be your decision and not your doctor's. So, please get informed. This is important! I hope you are still 'awake' when you are reading this. I would like to recommend some water to get your energy and focus back. LOL.

Let's look at first the experiences, not to mention the expertise of a 90-year-old physician, Dr. Gifford, M.D. He is one of Canada's sweetest and most sincere older doctors. He is claiming that after a heart attack, you don't need medications but rather anti-oxidants. Wow! Let's get really serious about this.

We need more than one perspective to stay alive or to be totally accurate, to not be killed. So, listen!

Oxidation is the real issue. Oxidation, when it comes to heart attacks? This is a new concept...you might be thinking.

So, Kangen Water®, this super antioxidant water should work, and does work, for prevention of heart attacks and it can also help together with diet in reversing the hardening of the arteries, lower your cholesterol, get you into shape... etc. It worked for Fred, my husband. He is off all four kinds of so-called 'heart medications' that were prescribed to him after he had some minor strokes, bell's palsy and a heart attack. Seven years have passed since he is taking no pills, not even aspirin and thank God, he is feeling great. He feels better than ever in fact. I hate to think how his kidneys would probably be blocked by now or who knows what else, if he'd stayed on the medication!

It is a fact that after more than three prescription pills, no one can tell what the interaction of those pills will be!

Maybe you don't believe me and you shouldn't! I am not a doctor remember? So, here we have a medical opinion directly from the lion's mouth. This is what Dr. W. Gifford-Jones, a graduate of the University of Toronto and Harvard Medical School has to say. He is doing everything at age 90 plus, to let people know about using anti-oxidants to heal after heart attacks.

"Alarm clock: Because every morning should begin with a heart attack."

UNKNOWN

LOL. I did not use an alarm clock since 1994 when I quit my job at the bank. It helped.

The 'scare tactic' implemented by some doctors after people have heart problems works so well that 90 percent of people remain on drugs for the rest of their lives. They have to deal with the consequences of those pills for the rest of their lives. Kidney failure is just one of them. What a shame! Dr. W. Gifford-Jones wrote in his book *"90 +, How I Got There"*: "Finally, I decided to bet my life on Linus Pauling. I believe his research more than I believe the money driven research of the pharmaceutical companies." When the good doctor followed his doctor's advice after a heart attack nearly killed him twenty-five years ago, he almost died. After that episode he decided to become his own doctor. This happened thirteen years after **Dr. Sidney Bush, an English researcher proved it beyond any doubt with before and after pictures (I just realized that this sounds like a detective novel) that high doses of vitamin C and natural lysine are not only able to prevent but reverse the hardening of the arteries.** Dr. Bush, (1929-2009) being an Optician, had a monumental finding. He had prescribed for patients being fitted for contact lenses 6,000 milligrams (mgs) of vitamin C, and 5,000 mgs of lysine. He then took pictures of the retina, the back part of the eye, the only area of the body where doctors can see arteries and a year later took a follow-up photo. Dr. Bush deserved the Nobel Prize in Medicine. But his research was completely ignored and has sadly collected dust in medical circles, which is not surprising. **Everything like this will be supressed and pushed under the rug by the 'system'.**

"It was apparent when you heard him talk about his research, that he did not suffer fools easily. He had a habit of telling them, and medical societies they were wrong!" says Dr. Linus Paulding who after winning two Nobel Prizes was also "not believed". Dr. Bush died this year in Spain at age 90. We can't allow him and his research to be forgotten. Dr. Linus Paulding (1901-1994), was an American chemist, biochemist born in Oregon, who published over 1,200 papers and books. I hope you noticed that all these three doctors lived a long life, longer than 90. They must have known something. Will you trust someone who is preaching about longevity who dies of a heart attack at age forty-five? I don't think so.

Wow. When I told in Court that I quit all the heart medications pushed on me because I learned and I know that heart disease is totally reversible, I was called 'crazy' by an infamous doctor (Dr. Albert Ross Deep) in front of a judge. I apologise for mentioning this monster's name

The Purple Wave

on the same page with these genuine doctors. Dr. Deep of Toronto, Ontario lost his Medical Licence, ten years after I tried to bring him to justice and lost $150,000 in the legal process. Thank God I refused the pills. [mostly beta blockers]. Three years later we found out that the diagnosis was wrong altogether and that I did not have heart disease (this was years before my hemi block discovery)! Imagine taking poisonous drugs for a condition you don't even have! Can things get crazier than that? I later found the root causes of chest pain and muscles spasms I was having; a buildup of heavy metals in my heart and other muscles and, of course, an extremely dehydrated body.

Getting back to Dr. Gifford now, he was so excited about this medical breakthrough that he wanted to talk about the Big Story and proven research data on National Television. He couldn't. He was stopped!

This is just one reason why you don't know about the real power of anti-oxidants. This is why you never heard about the real causes of heart problems. This is what I am talking about when I say that these things are suppressed by Big Pharma who owns the Media and, of course, most Governments are in bed with these two.

"Whoever controls the media controls the mind!"

JIM MORRISON

This is what Dr. Gifford said after he was stopped from telling the truth about heart disease and anti-oxidants on TV in Canada: "I'm mad as hell and I am not going to take it anymore ... I was commissioned to do a thirty second commercial on CBC ... but according to the 'rules' established by the Canadian Ministry of Health I could not say this product is helpful for the heart, only for the bones, teeth and gums, **when the product's main purpose is to prevent the nation's number one killer, heart attacks.** "So, why wouldn't this censure make me mad as hell?"

He further states, "Health Canada's regulation is a blatant distortion of scientific facts and a perfect example of thoughtless, bone-headed inconsistency." I personally think it's more than that. Much more. Okay, I am hesitant but I will say it. It is murder and that is not acceptable to me as a child of God. It will never be.

"Truth has a power only the courageous can handle."

ANTHON St. MAARTEN

Ladies and gentlemen, listen to these courageous doctors and scientists who speak up! No wonder most people are confused. This is just one example of how the system is working hard to confuse us. The attacks on good doctors are endless. That's why you never hear about the real solutions like vitamin 'C' or Kangen Water® when you're looking for an answer. **It doesn't matter if it's for prevention, wellbeing or longevity, these are good for you; it doesn't matter if it's your heart, or your brain, or whatever but doctors won't tell you that as they have to follow "the system".**

Genetics constitute only ten percent of the possibility of you living a long, healthy life or being ill. How you live is 90 percent. Please research Epigenetics, which will always override the 'gene theory'. Don't be fooled by thinking your genetics will sentence you to diseases your parents had. "Epigenetics' is the science or significant study and findings of changes caused by modification of gene expressions, rather than alteration of the genetic code," experts say. I hope you got it. In other words, it doesn't matter really what your genetics are saying, what you do with it (in other words, your lifestyle) will override those genetical parameters. For example, I inherited both heart and liver issues from my parents so I am genetically weak on both. Who cares? I used to think that I will die at the same time from the same issues as my parents did. Today I think different. My Mom died from the pills prescribed to her, not from the liver problem she inherited. She should have taken care of her sensitive liver and never taken any pills. She would still be here. This is what I am doing. I am completely clean of prescription pills. I have a Kangen® machine on my counter. I value and use vitamin C, the discovery of a brilliant man, mentioned several times before, whose name is on the 'black list' or something like that in North America, Dr. Albert Szent-Gyorgyi.

The Purple Wave

These are the stories and the details you need in order to get 'the big picture', I think. This is what made me see. When we are talking about Vitamin C, we are not talking about a pill a day, but 10,000, 15,000 or even 20,000 milligrams of vitamin C per day. These are very high doses. It is hard to stay on these or even pay for them. Many naturopaths work with these high doses. They are usually injected intravenously at special clinics as treatments for cancer patients. I did this when I did chelation to rid my blood of the heavy metals.

How much easier it is to drink super antioxidant water, which is 200,000 times stronger than vitamin C. You don't need needles nor do you need to spend thousands of dollars. A practical solution, a common-sense approach. We must multiply here by 6.9. You do the math! Find the oxidation reduction potential of Kangen Water® at -600 mV, compared to vitamin C, which is -100 mV. For me it is just wasting time, I just prefer drinking the water.

Dr. Gifford, Dr. Bush and Dr. Paulding are not the only doctors who know the truth about the heart and have the boldness to talk about it. There are many more. A world-renowned heart surgeon, Dr. Dwight Lundell, M.D. who is the past Chief of Staff of Surgery of a Heart Hospital in Mesa, Arizona, speaks out on what really causes heart disease and admits that they were wrong and have been saying the wrong things for a long time. Here we go, we just peeled another layer off the 'onion' of many lies. This was my mission from the beginning.

> *"Good God, no. The lies we tell other people are nothing compared to the lies we tell ourselves."*
>
> **DEREK LANDY**

Dr. Lundell states: "I trained for many years with other physicians labelled as opinion makers. Bombarded with scientific literature, continually attending education seminars, we 'opinion makers' insisted heart disease resulted from the simple fact of elevated blood cholesterol. The only therapy was prescribing medication to lower cholesterol and severely restricted fat intake. **Deviations from these recommendations were considered heresy and could result in malpractice."**

He further states: "We physicians with all our training and authority often acquire a rather large ego, that tends to make it difficult to admit, we are wrong. So, here it is, I fully admit to being wrong. Animal fats contain less than twenty percent omega-6 and are much less likely to cause inflammation than the supposedly healthy oils. Forget the science that has been drummed into your head for decades. Since we know that cholesterol is not the cause of heart disease, the concern about saturated fat is even more absurd today."

Here you have it again from the lion's mouth. What is causing all this inflammation in the body? Acidosis, which is caused by toxicity, and results in lack of oxygen which can be taken care of by proper hydration and detox. Oxidation the other big issue can be taken care of by antioxidants. Did you get it? Just another small piece of the puzzle, don't lose it! All this might be confusing to some. I understand, but we are at crossroads. A very important time in history, when you can shine if you are awake and understand what is going on. Our basic freedoms to choice, free speech and to be healthy and make the best decisions for ourselves is under attack and is going away. Time is up. We all have to speak up and defend our God given rights, so no corrupt billionaires, politicians and other evil creatures can harm our families and ruin our future.

Please let me recommend a TEDx talk on YouTube. This one is about the manipulation of the public. It is called, 'Astroturf and Manipulation on Media Messages," by Sharyl Attkisson. Great information and a 'must' watch for anyone. It will explain to you how far we have advanced in telling lies. We have professional liars who get paid to lie. What they say becomes more believable than truth! Then, of course, we need professionals who catch these lies. As long as everyone is making money! Just saying...

By eliminating inflammatory foods (the typical North American diet) drinks with sugar, processed everything and going back to origins, whole foods, fresh, unprocessed, normal, natural water and produce, you will reverse years of damage in your arteries. Beautiful and possible.

"Truth is not fully explosive, but purely electric.
You don't blow the world up with the truth,
you shock it into motion."

CRISS JAMI

The Purple Wave

Oh, I love real strength, power and skills, an invincible ability to shock things into motion. A great 'shock' is as good as pain is. I met many people in different countries where I lived who are scared of the truth. In their minds, truth is considered exactly that, something which might 'blow up' the world. They avoid shocks at any cost, if possible. It is a new trend nowadays. Let's be quiet and smile, make sure no one gets offended. Not me. Oh, I love truth more than anything on this Earth. Let's put things into motion with some truth and 'electric water'! These 'goodies' shouldn't be toxic or foreign to us, 'electrical beings'....

"The truth only hurts when you want to believe a lie."

JENNIFER McVEY

Ouch Jennifer, you said it not me.

CHAPTER 30

HER MEMOIR

"We are made wise not by the recollection of our past, but by the responsibility for our future."

GEORGE B. SHAW

We saw throughout the book how important drinking good water is. We found out how Enagic® reproduced nature's water and learned about the benefits of this truly functional water. I shared with you my story and how this water changed my life. I personally think that this miraculous 'renewal' or remaking of water comes with great responsibility. What if this is our last chance? Nowadays, 'responsibility' is a neglected word so let's put it back into our vocabulary!. We all should take responsibility. We have to analyse what has to be done and what our part is! We have to set the record straight. *"We have to be the change we want to see in the world."* This water is our source of energy and great health. It is our source of life and wellbeing. We have to 'govern ourselves accordingly'. I am using a 'legal term' intentionally as this issue is serious enough. We need more souls like Vandana Shiva. More courage and boldness. She hardly needs any introduction. Look her up on YouTube.

The Purple Wave

Environmental warrior and scientist Vandana Shiva (born in 1952) is an Indian scholar, environmental activist, food sovereignty advocate, and anti-globalization author who founded the Research Foundation for Science, Technology, and Natural Resource Policy (RFSTN), an organization devoted to developing sustainable methods of agriculture, in 1982. Her work is extremely important, when it comes to preserving our food supply. I love Vandana. Her boldness is admirable. She created a movement we all should be part of. She is brilliant and smart but more importantly she had the courage to stand up to one of the biggest global corruption of our time.

Another soul who understands the responsibility we have especially when it comes to water is Betsy Damon. I find what she does fascinating.

Please read a small section of Betsy's Memoir. You wont be sorry. She is a humanitarian whose work in the field of the art and science of water is significant. She has nothing to do with Kangen Water®, or Enagic®. Hers is yet 'another perspective', but wow, how similar our experiences are; hers with the spring water she found in nature and mine with Kangen®, which 'mimics' nature's water.

Betsy Damon has received over thirty awards and she is the founder of the 'Keepers of The Waters Foundation'. We can all learn from her experiences. She has worked with Eastern civilizations who seem to understand the relationship with water better than we do in the West.

I hope and pray that we, in the western civilizations, will also learn our moral responsibility toward protecting water and stick to them. We have a long way to go as we will have to go back and rebuild nature's way**, meanwhile we should do what we can to stop bottling water.** In my humble opinion, embracing the Kangen® device would be a great first step towards this noble mission. Again, Kangen Water® is 100 percent environmentally friendly.

There are a few marvellous lessons for all of us in Betsy's Memoir. She starts her story like this: *"In 1991 on the streets of Chengdu, I was asked to speak English with a group of Chinese professors. Among these professors was a biologist studying the health effects of water from a spring, called the 'God Water', twenty hours to the north.*

He had found that the waters reduced tumors in the mice and assisted in digestion. *My curiosity was sparked; I was determined to visit the 'God Water'."*

In this 'age of cancer', is your curiosity sparked yet?

She goes on: *"Alongside the spring sat a newly built pagoda where I was offered a drink of the water.*

I drank deeply and to my great surprise my body responded immediately with sensations that I have felt -a kind of aliveness in my cells.

Our guides told us that by local practice this water was only to be drunk, not used for cooking or washing. When the inhabitants of the area were ill, they would visit the Llama and for a small fee he would prescribe water...

People no longer had to pay for the water, now they could have it for free. We soon learned that the heap of broken glass bottles was there because glass was too heavy to transport down the mountain. **They began using plastic bottles only to discover that the waters lost the medicinal properties in a few days.** *I was witnessing that moment when a water source that sustains people's health is bottled up and sent to far-off places. The water is dislocated, becomes anonymous, and the people who have protected and relied upon this water for thousands of years are severed from their life source. The knowledge contained in these waters would soon be forgotten ... I have come to respect water as* **the most aggressive creative force** *we know."*

> **"I've given my memoirs far more thought than any of my marriages. You can't divorce a book!**
>
> **GLORIA SWANSON**

You too, Gloria? It is absolutely fantastic to know that I am not alone in this one. LOL.

Unfortunately, here in Canada (the land of abundant water reserves) the authorities don't really give a damn. Maybe because we still have water? As far as I know, the 'human relationship' with water in recent times has largely been characterized by neglect, control and exploitation by special interest groups, rather than celebrating, preserving, and acknowledging this essential element of life. This is more than depressing. I can't talk about this subject and not feel pain.

The Purple Wave

It is a much better idea to follow Betsy on her adventure: *"The visit to the 'God Water' propelled me forward. From the Living Water Garden, I went on to work in Beijing with many companies as a designer of 'living' systems. I witnessed the simultaneous elimination of historic water sites, and the development of the Olympic park with its vast wetlands and forests. I was proudly shown these historic water sites when I first came to Beijing, and when they were eliminated by development, there was an uproar. I witnessed a city that was caught between development, and their cultural history of honoring water...*

In cities around the world it is common practice to plan and build without understanding the available water. We 'transfer' more water. We dam more rivers. Springs and streams are built over, wetlands filled, intertidal estuaries are polluted or developed into precarious housing. **Rivers and their ecosystems lose their capacity to be resilient...**

This trip began my seven-year exploration of the water cultures in western Sichuan with a Tibetan filmmaker. We visited over forty different water sites, and found an extensive culture of honor and conservation throughout the Himalayas ...

On the mountain road to Muli Monastery is a small temple honoring a gushing stream. I was told that after the Cultural Revolution, with the extensive deforestation in the area, the stream had run dry. I asked the head monk how the water returned, and, with a grin, he said he replanted the forest. **He understood that the forest protected the waters.**

The people in these communities understood that the water was connected to the land and their actions, forests ensured springs would run, herd animals should stay away from headwaters, that human consumption should be thoughtful and moderate. They were keepers of their resources. When valued water sites are destroyed and the practices of respect and protection are abandoned, we lose an understanding of the essential connection between water and life. However, it is possible to build and design cities where the waters are collected, protected and celebrated, where everyone can thrive in cooperation with life-giving systems.

The water's right to be alive is inextricably linked with our right to life, and the right to life of all living forms."

The water should have the 'first right'. Giving this first right to water would be our responsibility. Wow, did you notice? She sounds like she is talking about Kangen water® when she, for the first time, experienced this healing spring water. What a validation for all of us by someone who has never tried or heard about Kangen Water®. This should make us think seriously about nature, our future, the next generation, health and preserving our marvellous resources. In this Memoir, I found the last piece of the puzzle I was looking for.

I am grateful for great humanitarians. Don't you love these initiatives, which **lead to life and total prosperity,** not only material profits? I am also grateful for Mr. Ohshiro and his 'disciples'.

The forests, the oceans and nature in general need our compassion, as much as people do, if not more. Thanks to our water generating machine we never have to use non-reusable plastic any more. We have more energy, "we feel a kind of aliveness", just like those who live near these sites in nature. We look healthier and we are happy for the many we are helping. These are the 'side effects' of this living water that we are enjoying so much!

We all desire a better world. We would like to see less pain and suffering, less misery. We need this ancient knowledge as much as we need modern technology and we need to live with love and compassion. **From science and technology, we should embrace only those ideas which will cause no harm!**

Half of the world's wetlands have been lost to development. The world's water is increasingly becoming degraded in quality, threatening our health and the ecosystems. The cost of fresh water is continuously increasing. The world **must return to its origin** when there were no poisons and plastic used. How do you think that will happen? I am sure that properly ionised water, 'the world's healthiest substance,' as Dr. Bob McCauley calls ERW will be part of it. Bob McCauley is a Certified Master Herbalist and a Naturopath Doctor. Herbalists understand nature and natural. Yes, Kangen Water® will be part of our future. It is here already. It has been implemented in our lifestyle for almost a decade and it's working!

"The doctor of the future will give no medicine but will interest his patients in the care of the human frame, in diet and in the cause and prevention of disease."

THOMAS EDISON

The Purple Wave

Yes, both the doctor of the past and the doctor of the future. We now live in the future Edison was talking about. Why wait? If we wait we will just experience more damage!

The Universe with its well established, unbeatable laws. Prevention, vitality, performance and happiness.. All the good stuff. A better future will arrive only with a better understanding of the past, when we had a higher moral code and a much more natural lifestyle.

CHAPTER 31

GENIUSES

*"Genius is talent set on fire
by courage."*

HENRY VANDYKE

There are many great thinkers in Europe, Japan, Korea and North America who are behind the science of Electrolyzed-Reduced-Water and there is a good reason why more and more doctors and scientists are coming on board.

I must mention that finally American scientists are also getting involved and excited about H2 and water.

According to modern day science (nowadays we can measure almost everything as we have marvellous technological instruments) the cells in the human body function normally around -20 to -22 mV but for the body to heal itself, it needs a minimum of -50 mV.

How much is an mV exactly? A millivolt (mV) is equal to one thousandth of a Volt.

When dehydrated, most people just don't have the extra voltage (energy) to heal. This is bad news. Here comes the problem. As your 'voltage'- your life force - goes down, you will get into the 'positive' and

The Purple Wave

in this case positive is very bad. Dr. Jerry Tennant, another expert states: "At +30 mVs, cancer cells turn on." Wow. Something to remember when we choose what we drink.

Please feel free to check out the work of another genius. Dr. Tennant is an M.D. who finished medical school in 1964 as top of his class at a University in Texas. In his book, "Healing is Voltage", he states: "Chronic pain always means low voltage. Illness begins when we can't make new cells". He explains that to make new cells we need the raw material, water being the main determinant and we need 'voltage'. Pesticides and other heavy metals, mercury, lead and poisons can interfere with this process. I find this quite simple and straightforward. Dr. Tennant thinks that everything is measurable. He is very impressed with Japanese technology. The Japanese are leading the world with their instruments. Nakatani, a well-known acupuncturist, can measure even the waves used in acupuncture.

So, we learned that we are electrical beings and healing is voltage. Now that you understand the concept, which one will you choose? As it happens often in life you have multiple choices: tap water, sodas, other beverages, bottled water, or anything else that measures between +300 and + 500 mV or Kangen Water®, which measures somewhere between -400 and -800 mV, depending on the source water. You don't have to tell me, just choose wisely.

Ok, let's talk about Hydrogen one more time. This is the fastest and easiest way to start getting better. This is self-recovery and self-healing at its best! Hydrogen also impacts cell signaling, cell metabolism, and gene expression because it is bioavailable and bio-dynamic.

What a fabulous miracle contained in water!

Hydrogen has been here from the very beginning. It makes sense, doesn't it? This is the theory, of course, but I experienced this in real life. Many times, when I have 'extra stuff' to get rid of like extra pollution, over eating, stress or frustration, tainted food' unwanted viruses or bacteria, I just double my water intake. It's quite easy to verify if the theory works by putting it into practice. You have to try the water! It works every time and you can take that to the bank.

> *"Simplicity is the most difficult thing*
> *to secure in this world; it is the last limit*
> *of experience and the last effort of genius."*

GEORGE SAND

I can only imagine the fight and politics between scientists today. Corrupt scientists must feel really threatened. They will deny this new discovery until they die.

This must be a huge slap in the faces of these hypocrites.

Synthetic versus Natural.

One has horrible side effects (pills) while the other (H2) is totally selective. Intelligence is built into it. It is estimated that 1600 scientists are presently researching Molecular Hydrogen worldwide.

Now you have it.

I hope you will never forget to drink - and to drink the right water. If not, well, I will tell you with great sadness that you can't be helped as nothing else will help you this much and this fast. It wasn't possible for me, either. We people are only happy if we are capable, if we have enough energy to perform well and really live and if we have a brain that works for our benefit.

We must have the great feeling of accomplishment to be happy most of the time. Many are lacking the extra energy required to be able to perform in life so please remember this always ... life starts with water (even in the womb)! Once you are properly hydrated, your brain will be comfortable, it will make the right decisions, it will help you to get off your butt! I witnessed this truth in the case of my daughter Eleonora who after becoming properly hydrated suddenly became active and started to do Stairs, Zumba and Yoga, after being a couch potato for a decade. Her mood also changed. She became a different person and no other change happened in her life when she replaced the sodas with Kangen Water®. It was a very happy time of my life when I saw all the positive changes in my family from this water. This 'life force' is needed before you go to the gym or even before you start socializing with people.

It is the first step to feeling whole or even human. Remember those one-time assets in the brain, the neurons (mentioned by Dr. Batman)? These are huge and valuable assets and we should take care of them.

Once they are damaged by lack of water, heavy metals, aluminum or chemicals, you will cease to exist as a human being. This is why dementia such as Alzheimer's and all neuro-degenerative problems should be prevented. Think about this before you accept the pills or eat foods with added chemicals. You can avoid huge problems with such little effort.

Once, not long ago I got 'vertigo'. It wasn't really vertigo; it turned out that chemicals were messing with my brain. The spinning and dizziness were unbearable. It was caused by baked goods I usually don't buy. Big supermarkets use specific (and dangerous) chemicals to keep the baked stuff 'fresh'. This poison apparently will cause dizziness. Thousands are wrongly diagnosed with "vertigo". Another label, which became popular lately. How do I know this?

Not long before this happened to me, I watched an eye-opening video with Peter Glidden. Dr. Glidden, ND, successfully worked with governments to get approval and licensing of Naturopathic Doctors as 'primary care' physicians. With 60 to 100 speaking engagements per year, Dr. Glidden is one of the most widely lecturing naturopathic doctors in the United States. He studied at the University of Massachusetts in Preventative Medicine. He is warning people on this video about these types of poisons in baked goods. This is how I realised what was happening to me. It was impossible for me to open my eyes. My brain was in such a crisis. My GOD. I honestly thought that it was over for me. Thankfully, after falling off my bed the morning after I ate this garbage (croissants), I could crawl to my phone. I called my husband who acted fast and brought me a glass of 11.5 pH water. This cleaned me out. Me, vomiting like crazy lasted a couple of hours. I doubled my 9.5 pH water intake and after three days I was better. Thanks to the water, I avoided hospitalisation once again.

"The reconnection of society, economy and ethics is a project we cannot postpone."

MICHAEL D. HIGGINS

Ethics, a 'project'? Being ethical for the benefit of society should be commonplace or the only way we operate. What are we doing? We are getting poisoned. We must stop this insanity somehow. We are using thousands of chemicals, even some which are banned in Europe and other countries. We are poisoning people for the sake of profit. If you eat garbage regularly, you won't be able to tell what is causing your dizziness or other symptoms and chances are you will be misdiagnosed and medicated. So, your 'chemical trauma' will be treated with more chemicals.

Do you remember the time when we used home remedies as we did not have pharmacies at every corner? The Kangen® machine is the new 'home remedy' in our house.

Dizziness is getting more and more common and it was non-existent thirty years ago when I started my insurance career. I never saw that in anyone's medical history. Now, I see it all the time! This makes me scream! Please eat fresh food from the market, if possible!

The big lesson I learned is that we really have to look after our brain as the rest of the body depends on it.

There are too many 'burned out' people who can't get out of the vicious cycle or take care of themselves, make good decisions or act in their own best interest. There are far too many who can't take care of their kids and family. I was blessed by Kangen Water®. As soon as I took care of myself, I could take care of my family members. The Kangen® machine is now in the home of many people I know.

This water is known and widely used by the different Presidents of the United States, and many exceptional athletes, even by some celebrities.

You might be wondering why U.S. presidents are drinking Kangen Water®? President Trump's energy and mental sharpness is hard to miss. (The stress, which comes with the office is not ordinary.) Here is the answer: This is what Dr. Gerald Bresnahan, M.D., the famous cardiologist to Presidents is saying. *"We have understood the importance of alkalizing diets for decades, but we have been unsuccessful in getting our patients to eat a perfectly alkaline diet. Hundreds of thousands of patients have seen remarkable results from drinking this therapeutic water. We are doing our part, in bringing this technology to the medical community in the United States because Kangen Water® is revolutionizing the health, fitness and wellness of our nation."* I am guessing this is why the presidents of the United States are drinking Kangen Water®! (Our poor Prime Minister, Mr. Trudeau, on the other hand, is showing signs of dehydration like brain fog, extreme confusion... etc.) *Klara, stop it! You promised that you won't*

The Purple Wave

'diagnose'. I might end up in jail but this was fun and hopefully it won't be interpreted as 'political'.

Are you up to date? All this is quite simple, all you need is a bit of Faith, or perhaps, some Curiosity!

As far as I am concerned, the dark days are over. We don't have to be presidents or billionaires to 'hack' our way to exceptional health.

We are discussing the biggest secrets of well being and the most updated information openly, aren't we? Besides, health and longevity are not supposed to be 'classified information'. We are done. Now your health is only up to *wonderful You.*

"The secret of genius is to carry the spirit of the child into old age, which means never losing your enthusiasm!"

ALDOUS HUXLEY

CHAPTER 32

PLACEBO?

"Experience is a hard teacher
because she gives the test first,
the lesson afterward."

VERNON LAW

I learned hard lessons through all these experiences, that's for sure. This is why when I meet a 'skeptic' I am confused. I am not sure if I should cry for them or laugh at them.

The skeptics can be stopped fast when we offer Kangen Water® to our pets or animals in general. They don't know what they are drinking, right? Still, it is documented by us and many other pet and horse owners that animals choose this water when they are given a choice. They love it; they drink more of this water and they also have tremendous results. (Remember Ely?) The 'placebo theory' is destroyed right away. Animals have no idea that they are given different water, yet, they have results and get healthier by drinking Kangen Water®. Dear skeptic [if you are still here], think about this for a while. In the meantime, I will tell you another story.

The Purple Wave

Our dog, Sky, went through a lot in his life: surgeries, infections, dangerous bacteria, allergies and so on. He should have been dead a long time ago. However, he was recently tested and he has no cancer or any other health issues. He is eight years old, which is already a nice age for a golden retriever. He was also 'mistreated' by a vet for a couple of years because of an ugly ear infection from a bacterium, which got under his skin, yet he is still full of energy just like a puppy. He survived four surgeries, which he needed because of the incompetence or the money grab of this vet. I am so tempted to say her name.

The reaction of animals to Kangen Water® completely annihilates the 'placebo theory'.

The next Kangen® machine I am buying will be donated to an institute in Romania where my younger brother has been for a few years now after suffering a brain injury as a child. I can't wait to see the results. I know it will help him. The miraculous effects of this water on brain inflammation caused by physical, even emotional or chemical trauma, has been seen many times. I see most vaccines as a great potential to cause a chemical trauma in the brain of a child. Autism is one of those horrible situations. We got 70 million autistic victims today. This has been proven time and time again, by data, statistics and the family members of these poor children and by other means. Now you can understand why molecular Hydrogen is extremely beneficial for kids with autism. Do you know anyone who has an autistic child? Autistic or healthy, make sure your child never sees a can of soda. They have to drink tons of water.

I hope I answered most of your questions about this phenomenon. The medical device called the Kangen® machine is the most valued appliance in our family by far. We would not take vacations without it. Who wants misery during a nice vacation? It will help you to avoid emergency rooms, drug stores, hospitals, lineups, dealing with mosquito bites or other nasty insects, unnecessary spending and wasting money on plastic water. The uninformed person will not survive in today's environment. This is why our work is important and is indeed a huge opportunity to make the world a better place.

The big difference between us and other companies is this; Enagic® is not willing to pay anyone for endorsements. Please check that out by all means!

A hundred years ago, usually only old people had strokes or blood clots, now younger and younger people are affected. We are dehydrated at a younger age as we have replaced water for the entire population with all sorts of marketed drinks. Anything goes these days, except natural, old-fashioned water.

To provide people 'dead' water which is not functional, it doesn't make any more sense than taking away fat from people who doubled their weight by eating sugar. There are no signs unfortunately that refined sugar will be taken away from society, no matter how bad it is.

One can have amazing water or even a Kangen® machine available but by looking at it only, they won't get hydrated.

> ### *"You can't cross the sea merely by standing and staring at the water."*
>
> **RABINDRANATH TAGORE**

We need to drink natural, 'normal' water! Why are we drinking water? Not for the taste as water has no taste. It should not have taste. If water had taste, it could not be 'universal' meaning that it would be loved only by those who like that taste.

There is a good reason why water has no taste.

It is for everyone. Period. We should taste wine and *drink* water. Instead we taste water and drink all sorts of alcohol and other beverages, often too much wine. We are doing it backwards. So, if we don't drink it for the taste, what are we drinking it for?

We need it for what it does, precisely for its main functions in the body, which once again are: to hydrate, to detoxify, to alkalize, to transport nutrients and to stop oxidation. Oops! These are the main causes of chronic illnesses. Dehydration, toxicity or acidosis, malnutrition and oxidation.

Now you can easily see that the benefits of Kangen Water® **coincide with the root causes of chronic illness. They are exactly the** **same.** This revelation was mind blowing to me. So, Dr. Batman, Dr. Lenkei and the rest of these amazing souls are right, they are not crazy. ***We are*** ***not sick, we are thirsty!*** This is the most logical and beneficial conclusion there is.

The Purple Wave

This is where the essence of therapeutic water is. There is no 'miracle' here. Everything is exactly as it should be. We fixed the water and it is drinkable again. More than that, it is working again.

How simple and how wonderful. You see, you only needed a tiny bit of help.

You needed to see the 'Big Picture'. Is there anyone who is not happy about this?

I sincerely hope that the 'characters' of this story, the Creator of Water, the doctors, the Nobel Prize winners, the geniuses like Albert Szent-Gyorgyi or Avicenna and Jerry Tennant, the scientific experts, the honest researchers, the people with testimonies including myself, we restored your Faith in Water.

"Any intelligent fool can make things bigger,
more complex, and more violent.
It takes a touch of genius-and a lot of courage
-to move into the opposite direction."

F. SCHUMACHER

Are you one of those people who lack courage? Does all this make sense to you now? Which 'direction' are you moving to? **Are you realising the most amazing reality that everything we need is available and it was given to us? We don't have to 'make' it ourselves!**

Your health is your choice. At least, it should be. My main concern is that the next generation has not much of a choice.

My first conclusion from all of this is that we can't have cellular health or health in general if we don't drink water, which is adequate in that regard. My second conclusion is that nowadays we are exposed to so many chemicals (like never before) that our bodies can't deal with it so we have to flush them daily and get used to this new lifestyle. It is not hard. It truly isn't. Especially if you love the water you are drinking.

The amazing idea of ionised water has caught the attention of many doctors, scientists, and users like myself, biologists, chiropractors, nutritionists, brain experts, and the whole world of the natural wellness and beauty industry. The strange part is that while one might be drinking plenty of regular water, one is not getting properly hydrated and definitely not getting results. This is because of the lack of absorption or the broken structure of bulk water.

Another thing I learned is that the one common denominator of all chronic conditions is acidosis. This is great news, I think, in the sense that we only need to care about one thing and not worry about many different conditions. Some say, "Oh, it doesn't matter what I do to look after myself because if I don't die of cancer or Alzheimer's, I will die of a heart attack or a stroke, or something else. How can I protect myself from all those things? It seems like too much work to do." How naïve this kind of thinking is!

I hope that this long analogy (my apologies) brought you closer to understanding what we mean when we call the Kangen® machine, The 'Deal of the Century' the 'future of medicine', the 'ultimate solution', the 'purple wave', a 'tsunami', a new trend, 'peace of mind', a paradigm shift or the 'amazing health machine'.

When I first saw a Kangen Water® presentation, that unforgettable 'demo' by Roger Gaudette, I purchased the device right away. I didn't buy it for the drinking water as I did not know at the time that I would love this water and drink it. I also had no idea that arthritis and gout would ease up and all that crazy pain I had would go away.

The 11.5 pH water, which is so practical and potent when it comes to cleaning our produce from pesticides is what sold me the machine.

When I saw that I can easily remove herbicides and chemicals, I knew I'd found gold. 'Blue' Gold, which in fact is much more precious than 'yellow' gold!

Cooking with these waters and eliminating chlorine and other additives -cleaning the food properly - is a totally fantastic experience. Yes, my cooking is so tasty that I don't use any, I mean *any* spices or taste enhancers except sea salt and some fresh herbs. I use black pepper only if I prepare meat. Yes, Fred is a meat lover. Please know that if you don't soak your veggies and fruits in something like 11.5 pH water (there is nothing like this out there), you are poisoning (or letting others poison) your family and shortening the lives of your kids and grandkids...

When I was still living in Europe (approximately 50 years ago), America and Canada sounded like a safe place, a great place to immigrate to. Who knew that in 50 years time things would get this horrible? The astronomical amount, which is spent on health care, the $ 2.7 trillion won't take us far. 1.8 million people will be diagnosed with cancer in 2019, according to the American Cancer Society. The incidence of some cancers is on the rise including childhood cancers, leukemia and testicular cancer. We're experiencing a cancer epidemic and evidence is growing ever stronger that pesticide exposure is a key contributor to this disturbing trend. It's become a shared part of our culture. More than 600,000 men, women and children die from cancer each year, only in the United States, leaving millions of grieving siblings, parents and children behind. The situation is pretty much the same here in Canada and all over Europe.

"You beat cancer by how you live, why you live and in the manner in which you live!"

UNKNOWN

Entire industries have arisen to cope with the side-effects of cancer treatment as patients and their families struggle to live "normal" lives and enterprising businesses rush to fill the need. It's unclear exactly how much of cancer results from exposure to cancer-causing chemicals but the linkage has been significantly underestimated. Even before kids are born, they are bombarded continually with combinations of these dangerous exposures.

"I observed this again and again: During detox the tumor shrinks. During more exposure to toxins the tumor grows. "

DR. CHRISTIAN GONZALES
[Holistic cancer therapist, Naturopath doctor]

This is not the 'free' North American life I was dreaming about when I was growing up. There is no freedom in fear and suffering. I am sorry for being negative but I just had to say it. At the Abbotsford Cancer Centre here in BC, 70 percent of cancer patients are farmers of all ages and workers in agriculture. I saw this with my own eyes. Back home, 50 years ago, farmers were very healthy people! The last 50 years should never have happened. In 50 years, we 'arrived'. We are transforming the food we eat from nourishing, wholesome natural foods into poisonous, 'food-like' chemicals. This is the difference between the lifestyle of your grandfather (you know, the one who smoked all his life and died happily at age 93) and your child.

I am not sure how we can exercise enough pressure on the governments and politicians to do something about the immediate withdrawal of these poisons from our agriculture. In the meantime, we 'old-fashioned' women who are preparing wholesome food at home, we all embraced the 'Kangen Lifestyle'. We are washing a good chunk of these poisons out with our 11.5 high alkaline water but, of course, nothing is 100 percent.

We are ahead of the curve; we did not want to wait. Hopefully you can also see it with this "pandemic" or "Plandemic" [you decide, but please do your homework and get educated about the truth before you make this decision] that this became even more urgent for all of us. We happen to think that it's important to avoid not only premature death, hospitalization, 'ventilators', but strokes, wheelchairs, oxygen tubes, bypass surgery, chemotherapy, knee replacements, brain surgery and all the misery that comes with it.

I made my case, at least I think I did. I would like to see you on this journey and talk, if possible. In the meantime, I am wishing you great health and happiness, a pain-free life. You are worthy! You are a precious human being, a creation made in the image of God. You should be more like a magnificent stallion, which smells the water before it drinks it, not a donkey, which cannot tell the difference between a dirty pond or the crystal-clear water of a waterfall.

We should never compromise when it comes to truth and health.

"The kind of beauty I want most,
is 'the hard-to-get' kind that comes from
within- strength, courage, dignity."

RUBY DEE

CHAPTER 33

WATER BOOM

*"It is the sweet, simple things of life,
which are the real ones after all."*

LAURA I. WILDER

Imagine a group of people living together. At one point something goes wrong. A person is found dead and it's not a 'natural death', the person was killed. Without any investigation 'The Killer' is named but an innocent person is blamed. The chaos causes panic and soon new dead bodies start popping up. The situation will get worse and the problem will not be solved until the *real killer* is found.

I understand that this is a weird comparison but it feels like something similar is happening with our sick care system. A horror story is developing.

During the last thirty years since I began studying holistic health, I have seen the medical establishment blame many different things for our collective ill health: genes, germs and pathogens, family history, salt, fat, sugar, meat, milk, eggs, alcohol, tobacco, stress, extra weight, even the Sun.

There is nothing like life experience, friends. Life and suffering taught me that these might be factors to a certain point. 'The big animal' however, is none of these things. I am here to spread the word and make you aware about the two things that override all these things causing unprecedented damage when it comes to human health.

Gradual cellular dehydration is the main cause. Dr. Batmanghelidj summed it up by saying, *"Genes are not cast-iron structures. They must be replicated from raw materials that are carried by water circulation in the body. Since the body, except the neurons that are one-time assets of the brain, remakes itself every so many weeks, every genetic abnormality that is seen in later years, must be assumed to be initially the result of dehydration that became established some time before."*

Let's read further and see what is happening; ***"Today, these same diseases are blamed on the genetic makeup of the people. If medical professionals would only realize that the 'drought' in the internal environment of cells in the body impacts the enzymic activity of the DNA and RNA structures of the nucleus of the cells! Thus, most of the malfunctions of these genes is secondary to the missing action of water in the interior of the cells."***

Isn't he brilliant? So, yes, lack of water would be number one.

Number two derives from number one naturally. The root of the problem is not found; therefore, the wrong 'treatment' is implemented. This uninvited interference destroys the body further. Now the body must deal with new poisons, as well. I am surprised that we are not dying even faster.

When I was so ill that I could hardly function, I started to cry in the middle of a health food store. A nice clerk came my way and asked me what the problem was. All I could say to her was that there was nothing I could eat that wouldn't make me sick. I blamed the food. When I visited a few doctors, they told me that it was all in my head. They blamed my mental state and some of them offered me pills. When I went to different holistic healers, they helped me a bit, and I paid a lot but, in the end, it was lack of water, lack of essential minerals (because of lack of water) and everything these things caused that was hurting me most. No one ever mentioned water or proper hydration to me before I found the 'Kangen Family'. Who are they? They are all those people who have the light; they realised what good water can do for them. They have a different mindset from the rest of the people.

The Purple Wave

> *"There is a hidden message in every waterfall.*
> *It says, if you are flexible, falling will not hurt you!*
>
> **MEHMET MURAT ILDAN**

Today, it is a different life for me. I am managing my body and health, mostly with this therapeutic water. I am a new person. I rebuilt my immune system and guess what? Miraculously, I can now tolerate a normal, natural diet. Guess what else? I don't get injured, no matter how much I exercise. Here I am, giving you another big secret. Never start gym, fitness, exercise of any kind before you hydrate yourself well at the cellular level. This secret will help you to avoid tons of injuries.

After forty-five years I got my life back.

This is what I call: Winning the battle!

> *"There are two educations. One should*
> *teach us how to make a living,*
> *and the other, how to live."*
>
> **JOHN ADAMS**

When I was feeling unbelievably horrible and the itchiness was driving me crazy, the fatigue was simply paralysing, my muscles were weak and the spasms were killing me ... when it felt like I couldn't take it anymore and the chest pain did not go away for a month ... finally then and only then, I, the 'Avicenna' of this century asked: Why? What is the cause? I was told it is 'psoriasis' and 'fibromyalgia' and a few other ailments. "We are not sure," they said. I said, "Yes, but there must be a reason!" and they said, "Oh, yes, it is in your head." I knew that wasn't it! Then I realized that I am craving sugar all the time and I am eating sweets like there was no tomorrow (I actually 'had to eat' a whole, big-size mango cake from a Chinese bakery in my car as soon as I paid for it in front of TD-Canada Trust on Finch Ave in North York, Ontario). One cannot forget about something like this. When this happened, I knew I was in deep trouble! Why do I have these cravings? I asked myself and I researched it. It is Candida, you silly. Candida? What is Candida? I wanted to know. When I got shingles, I asked again, "Why?" Then I found this out; my immune system is 'down'. Why is my immune system down? I realised I was over-acidic from all the sugar and everything else. Yes, of course, I am acidic, but how did I get here? Because I am toxic. Yes, but why so much toxicity? Dr. Ewing, a wonderful Naturopath doctor from Abbotsford, BC (the clerk from the health food store sent me there), told me that I was poisoned. How come? I was poisoned with mercury and lead, he said. Why? Then, I opened my mouth and he found eight amalgam fillings from 'cheap' (mainstream) dental work. The story ended when he got those out and I did the treatment which financially bankrupted my family. It took about two years and tonnes of money, for me to rebuild my immune system.

"I have no special talents. I am only passionately curious."

EINSTEIN

Twenty-three or so years later, I found the answer. Why did this happen to me when so many have amalgam in their mouths? Finally, after reading and learning about chronic cellular dehydration (flushing the cells, drinking water) it clicked in.

The main cause why the heavy metals almost killed me was, yes, chronic involuntary cellular dehydration!

This is how "I carried my life" without water.

What happened in the last seven years is my personal encounter with Kangen Water®. I don't want to keep you up all night with endless testimonials, I am sure by now, you got the idea. The next chapter could never happened without the water. When we are truly alive we can do amazing deeds many things which seemed impossible before.

CHAPTER 34

FREED BY RESTRICTIONS?

"Don't ask what the world needs.
Ask yourself what makes you come alive
and then do that. Because what the world
needs is, people who have come alive."

HOWARD THURMAN

There are too many who yet need to "come alive" and yes, the world really needs them. I love this affirmation filled with wisdom and hope. Many are not really free. I wasn't free myself until not long ago. I still felt bound by some kind of stranglehold even after drinking the water for eight years. How come? I am glad you asked. Well nothing but, the food I was accustomed to kept me captive. A very restricted new diet freed me which I know it sounds weird but it is the absolute truth.

I should name this Chapter, *"The 90 days which made me come physically totally alive and free"* or something of that sort but that would sound like a commercial. The story I need to tell you is not an ad, a sales pitch or anything of that sort. It is completely personal, almost embarrassing. So, how to really come to life if you live in this era of fear, sickness, tainted foods, poisons and addictions. Yes, there are many 'land mines' but there is a huge difference between danger and fear. One is real, [danger] the other one is a fiction, a lie, an imaginary or scary agent. Yes, I think that is how I would define fear. Many are paralyzed by it, as they don't differentiate between fear, which is quite ridiculous and real danger. Is it possible, to achieve complete freedom? This will add an entire chapter to this story, but my personal testimony as a life-long 'patient' would not be complete and totally true, if I would not mention this.

What you heard to this point was my so-called 'dehydration story' only. Now we will talk about something quite different. This additional story, my so called 'starvation' story is again the true testimony of a woman who has an amazing appetite, access to almost any foods, money to buy it and some accumulated knowledge about health. She was malnourished as well, not only dehydrated and about 50 lb overweight. I am talking about silly me again, of course. You did not see this coming, did you? Well, you thought that I will be satisfied with just getting hydrated? I don't think so. If I got this far, I also wanted to be well nourished, and lose some more weight. I wanted all. To become 'ageless' required a bit of extra work. Yes, I know that I am crazy. That is me, Klara with a "K".

> **"If you approach the ocean with a cup, you can only take away a cupful. If you approach it with a bucket, you can take away a bucketful."**
>
> **RAMANA MAHARSHI**

I wanted to be *completely* healthy and avoid the danger that maybe I will eventually get cancer like my mom did at this age, or have a heart attack like my dad had at exactly this age. I never stopped reading and learning, observing what is going on around me. I came a long way, but not all the way. My weak heart is working quite well with the water, but I was sure that my addiction to foods and sugar, the constant cravings and over-eating sooner or later will jeopardize that. I had to finish the journey. Some loose ends made me go and have a couple of examinations

The Purple Wave

by professionals who have the real tools to see what is going on in the body at a cellular level. Oh no, I am not talking about X-ray, CT scan or, MRI. We want to go to the root causes remember? Again, why to spend time and money on a 'dead-end' diagnosis with no solutions? We want to prevent that tumour which has to be big enough so it can be detected by these harmful X-rays. This is why I like to use Live Blood analysis, Iridology and other methods to find out about my 'biomarkers', see how I am really doing. This again, is not just about me. Many of you are in the same situation. Yes, you might be malnourished or starving and you don't know it. You might be toxic, and you don't know why. We are what we **utilize,** not what we eat, I remembered. I had questions and I needed answers. I wanted to know about any new ideas and discoveries, just to make sure I am not missing anything as I did not see anyone for eight years.

This is the place and the time when we will to talk about nutrition, the remaining 25% of our diet. Yes, but which diet? There are thousands out there. What can we do for a diet in 2020 to avoid or prevent huge problems?

> **"The second day of a diet is always easier than the first. By the second day, you're off it."**
>
> **JACKIE GLEASON**

Okay, let's get serious. We should always start with "The Elimination Diet". First we must remove anger, regret, worry, resentment, guilt and blame. Immediately after these should be easier to remove sugar and junk all together. Wait! After letting you know that you are not hungry but thirsty, please allow me one more secret. You are not hungry. You are bored! When you learn the difference again it will be easier to do the right diet. This part was crucial to me. Oh boy, finally we got to the nutrition part of our diet plan.

There is a huge variation of foods out there. We all have different metabolisms, very different life styles and situations, different needs when it comes to diet. Nutrition is a science and an art, all in one. It is the best chemistry there is and the only chemistry we should have. When I tell people that I am on a very restricted diet, they immediately think I am 'vegan'?! Veganism is huge now a days, but vegan does not necessarily mean healthy or nutritious, I am sorry. You can avoid all meat, dairy or any animal product but you might eat a bunch of GMO grains, or meat substitutes that come from only God knows where. You might eat a bunch of white rice and other dead foods which are lacking enzymes for example. There is more, much more to nutrition than being a vegan or a vegetarian. There are some common denominators however, when it comes to what is good or bad to eat, but what might be okay for you can be bad for me. It is true, that foods can kill us and foods can heal us. Dr. Shinya who is a huge fan of Kangen Water® of course, on the front cover of his famous book: "The enzyme factor" has a subtitle which reads: *"Diet for **the future** that will **prevent** heart disease, **cure** cancer and **stop** Type 2 diabetes." This is the diet I need to tell you about.* This is the diet you might need even if it would not be your first choice. This is the diet I am interested in. Not keto, not trendy diets, not what a typical dietician might recommend. Have you noticed? He doesn't say treat, experiment, label, diagnose or something of that sort. He is using bold, powerful words, like **Prevent, Cure, Stop!** Now, why should we be listening to this man, and the many others who are all saying the same thing, like Dr. Matt Lederman, MD, Dr. Neal Bernard, MD, or Dr. Siu mentioned before? Perhaps we should listen to Dr. T. Colin Campbell, who authored the famous book everyone should read: "The China study". Oh, wait a minute, he is saying the very same thing the other four doctors and my amazing nutritionist, Ariel are saying. Let's see, what that is about...

Dr. Shinya states five or six times in his book that his patients who follow his diet have zero reoccurrence of cancer. Who can claim such a thing? Zero reoccurrence. Zero means none, zip, not one, not any. How is this possible? How can we believe this? I have to remind you that this doctor has been "watching" the entire gastro intestinal track and its characteristics, the 'microbiome' for about 50 years. [where all disease is starting!]

The most interesting thing I found about diet is this; In 1977 [45 years ago!], an interesting report about food and health was published in the USA. This was needed because health care costs started rising, putting enormous pressure on the economy. Despite the huge advancements in the medical field an enormous number of people were getting ill with cancer and heart disease and the numbers were going up year by year. The experts needed to draw a 'health plan' to combat this new trend, as the situation was getting out of hand and unsustainable. Top medical and nutrition specialists by collecting data from all around the globe came up with very clear results:

The 5,000-page 'summary' called The McGovern Report concluded that this situation with cancer and heart disease is a *direct consequence* of wrong dietary habits. Ok, so what are we doing wrong? Here it is. The food we eat not only feeds our cells, but also determines what kind of inner garden we are growing in our guts. This garden is filled with bugs that determine more about your health and your emotional and mental wellbeing than you ever imagined! Getting your gut bacteria healthy is one of the most important things you can do to get and stay healthy. If your 'bacteria' are sick, so are you! The foundation of a healthy gut begins with what we eat. We should focus on fiber-rich vegetables, greens, seeds and nuts, fresh whole fruits, different kinds of beans and legumes. This is exactly what I started to do. Our gut wall houses 70 percent of the cells that make up our immune system. Gut health literally affects our entire body. Consider the important jobs your gut performs regularly, including breaking down food, absorbing nutrients, keeping out toxins and producing nutrients. That's a lot of work! For optimal immunity, detoxification and nourishment, our gut must function seamlessly. The gut also houses 500 species, [three lbs] of bacteria. A growing field of research now focuses on the microbiome, called the second genome, and how it contributes to weight, disease and health. Too many bad gut flora (including parasites, yeast or bad flora) or not enough good bacteria can spell serious trouble for your health and your waistline. This is exactly what we discovered in my case. Yeast, parasites, starving cells, etc. Gut bacteria thrive on what you feed them, I learned. Some crazy scientists are talking about fecal transplants (infusing someone's poop into you) for weight loss. This is how important it is. An easier and more normal approach would be if we would feed our own bacteria by eating the right foods. I prefer to fertilize my own inner garden. If we eat fresh, real, natural, organic foods, the good bacteria will thrive. Eating 'junk', highly processed foods, bad fats, dairy, breads, yeast, alcohol and baked goods, we will have a leaky gut, and inflammation. The good news is that our microbiome changes with every bite of food, so we can positively alter our gut flora beginning with the very next meal.

Eating meat and animal protein often, will accelerate aging and will cause cancer and/or heart disease. Wow! Quite simple. Which part is hard for us to understand? The problem is that we are confused and we got accustomed to bad habits, useless traditions, restaurants and fast food places, cheap meat prices, easy and speedy cooking, BBQing, etc. What else to eat before we drink that great tasting cold beer, which looks so desirable? The problem is that what is not really natural for humans to eat in the first place became second nature for most of us. This is what makes us sick. No labels. Only two words: cause and effect, or cause and consequence. We are going to quickly learn the basics what we need to know about diet in 2020 and how to find the foods we can eat... Sorry, if I overwhelmed you with information, but this is really key to our health.

"Learning never exhausts the mind."

LEONARDO DA VINCI

Everything changed. *"What was okay to eat before 1980, it's not okay to eat it today"*, says Ariel Jarvis, my amazing nutritionist. Ariel is a Certified Herbalist and has a Ph.D. in Nutritional Sciences. She is the owner of Vitality Wellness Centre in Langley, BC. Wait a minute! Not to eat what we are so familiar with or we ate all our lives is quite an outrageous statement. Many won't like it, but that is not going to affect the truthfulness of it. I was as shocked as you are, to tell you the truth, but I realised the importance of it. Do you ever wonder, if there are people who know enough about nutrition and if they would reveal it to us? Is there anyone who can help us? Does anyone have such a complete knowledge and is it accessible by ordinary people like you and me? I assure you that they are out there. We have to find those individuals. I am glad I found a couple.

I know that mostly we create our health situation and our happiness.

"I have found that if you love life,
life will love you back."

ARTHUR RUBINSTEIN

The Purple Wave

I decided to stop the non-sense of not eating right. From now on I will definitely 'eat to live' and not the other way around. I have a lot to live for and things to do, I have to be healthy. I made a decision, a very hard one I must say. Restoring my heart health as much as possible, detoxing my liver, taking care of Candida overgrowth, loosing the extra fat, easing up my joints from the unnecessary pressure, taking care of digestion, absorption and enzymes, getting rid of more heavy metals, balancing my blood sugar, took a bit of work and some discipline but needless to say it was well worth it. I did all this in 90 days. I did this very same diet in 1994, and again in 2015 but only did it for a month and only lost about 30% of what I needed to. It worked then, and it worked again now. At the time, I was too isolated, to busy with too many things, so I did not stay with it. Big mistake from my part. **"Proper nutrition is the foundation of health, not genetics;"**- So many experts are pressing this and sharing the same opinion that we have to pay attention to it. There is definite truth in this idea. This is also called the "mucus free" diet. As a patient I can tell what is working well for me. This is not just reading something and deciding to believe it or not. This is real and it is working perfectly.

120 days after starting this protocol I can truly say that I am not only hydrated but also nourished. I am 'self made' and I am free of my food addiction. I can feel it, I can almost touch it. It is marvelous to be free.

"The self is not something ready-made,
but something in continuous formation
through choice of action."

JOHN DEWEY

There are many doctors who think that 'candida', the overgrowth of Candida Albicans is the precursor of cancer. In case of heavy metals this condition is quite common. To stop this yeast from killing you, one needs a mucus free diet, which is restricted, to say the least. I know that I am not alone in this. Functional medicine doctor, Dr. Amy Myers, MD claims, that "nine out of 10 patients she sees suffer from Candida overgrowth". Once you have a suppressed immune system by heavy metals you have to do the right thing for the rest of your life, if you want to live. Prevention is so much easier than any treatment. It is the smart thing to do. Yes, you need to pay attention and invest in a good diet, but again, what is the alternative? Chemo? Death? We deserve better.

> **"What is called genius is the abundance of life and health."**
>
> **DAVID HENRY THOREAU**

I am hearing it every day that people are going vegan. Why do you think that is? They have no choice if they want to enjoy life. People can tell that they are not well when they eat dairy and meat. Dr. Campbell in his book tells the story: *"A pattern was beginning to emerge: nutrients from animal-based foods increased tumour development, while nutrients from plant-based foods decreased tumour development."* Dr. Thomas Campbell, M.D. and Colin Campbell PhD. are the authors of the most comprehensive study about nutrition ever conducted. The unchangeable and unchallengeable truth is that you are not only what you eat, but what the animals you eat, are eating. What the animals are fed with today is very different from what they were fed with 50 years ago.

I had to make a decision. I wasn't digesting animal-based foods, meat and dairy all together. I depleted my "bank of enzymes" and the undigested food made me toxic destroying my intestinal flora. These toxins were making me bigger and bigger at my waistline. Large deposits of fat were needed to be created by my body around my waste line to store these poisons. There was no other way around it and there will never be. This is how the body functions and protects itself from sudden death caused by these toxins.

"An enzyme is a generic term for a protein catalyst that is made within the cells of living things. Wherever there is life, enzymes always exist." -states Dr. Shinya. More than 5,000 kinds of enzymes are created in the cells of our bodies. Currently enzymes are attracting significant attention globally as one of the key elements controlling our health. We did not hear about enzymes 50 years ago. Dr. Edward Howell a pioneer in enzyme research states: *"The number of enzymes a living thing can make during its lifetime is predetermined."* He calls this "enzyme potential"

The Purple Wave

and when this potential is stopped by the body, life ends. Interesting theory. Although all research on this is only in its developmental stage, Dr. Shinya is saying that; *"Abundant clinical evidence already exists showing that we can tremendously strengthen our gastrointestinal characteristics - and thus our health- by following diet that supplements enzymes and by mastering a lifestyle that doesn't exhausts the source 'enzyme'."* By talking to my nutritionist doctor and reading on this, I understood the importance of eating the right diet. Deep down in my heart I know that yes, indeed I am paying now for eating to much meat during the first 40 years of my life. This is the main reason I don't have any enzymes left, I think. Now by eating the right foods I don't overeat and I supplement with the required enzymes. This made all the difference. After 120 days eating delicious and wholesome foods I personally prepared, I lost the exact weight I wanted to lose. I achieved my goal by absolutely not trying to lose weight. I am very excited about the 'new me'. This time I am sticking with it, I feel so great. I tried this for far to long failing again and again. I did lots a 'yo-yo' dieting when I was younger, especially after a doctor pushed beta blockers on me for six months and I gained weight because of those meds. My situation was even worse, as all this extra fat was at my waistline, around the major organs. To get rid of this was a lot of fun and easy with the right diet. I got excited and the days just went by. No turning back from here dear friends. Yes, at age 65 I had to learn how to succeed on a plant-based diet and make things work without any grains except Quinoa. Piece of cake with great water. The only difficult period was the first two weeks. Now, that I lost all that weight, I am going to buy some new clothes and shoes. 'High hills' to be exact. Oh yes. Just because I am 'ancient old', it doesn't mean that I have to look like a cadaver.

"Success consists of going from failure to failure with no loss of enthusiasm."

WINSTON CHURCHIL

The lesson is this: If you are over eating or you can't stop eating – if you are always hungry or overweight - chances are that you are not nourishing yourself as either you are eating the wrong foods or you are not digesting effectively. Real natural foods are not addictive. It is all you, who is trying to get the satisfaction from food-like junk or tainted foods. Those are not nutritious and your body is not satisfied, nor will it ever be. You might be feeding the "Candida invaders" and not your cells. I know I did. The cravings stopped as soon as I dropped the foods which had no dietary fibres, no enzymes, or anti-oxidants. Cheeses and meats are in this category. Oatmeal and most of the other grains are not good for my heart either - I learned. Corn and white potato are off the table as well. I finally figured it out with the help of an amazing nutritionist, who is actually living what she is teaching and looks gorgeous. I realised that I don't need these foods, nor can I digest them any more. They were making me toxic, fat and unhappy. It is very smart to re-evaluate one's diet after age 55 or so.

This is how real freedom came to me after thirty-three years to be exact. It did not come when I first put my feet on the 'land of the free' many years ago, it only came now, in the year 2020.

"In the truest sense, freedom cannot be bestowed; it must be achieved."

FRANKLIN D. ROOSEVELT

I am very grateful for the wonderful recipes and for those new, great tasting foods I can eat now. The selection is huge. We just have to focus on the foods we can eat and not on those which we shouldn't. Thankfully there is an abundance of wholesome foods out there like nuts, seeds, legumes, fruits and vegetables, beans and lentils, okra and avocado, chickpea, and much much more. A whole new word opened up in front of me and I am seeing it now.

Why I am so much happier? Well, there is a two way communication between the gut and the brain, I learned. Dopamine, stress hormone and other signaling molecules are all produced in the gut. Attention people with mood disorders, depression, anxiety. When 'dysbiosis' occurs, an imbalance in the got, we are paving our way to a leaky gut, we feel miserable, and we are putting our immune system on fire. We need more anti-oxidants, more nutrients and more water, more of the good stuff. We

The Purple Wave

can have malabsorption even with good water and a good diet, if we lack enzymes and dont colonize the digestive track with enough good bacteria. A good selection of these can only be achieved in todays environment with a high quality probiotic. There was lots of new knowledge available on this front and I almost missed it again. I had to start to consume a quality probiotic daily, more fiber, lots a chlorophyll. Fermented foods are also amazing, Thank God for sauerkraut. I completely dropped all the sweets I used to eat, and I replaced wine with living water. I had no choice. Nothing is good for me which feeds Candida. No results without sacrifice. I am sure I heard that before. Now I am finally there. The love of freedom makes you do strange things I guess....

CHAPTER 35

WHERE EVERYTHING STARTS

*"If more of us valued food and cheer
and song above hoarded gold,
it would be a merrier world."*

J.R.R. TOLKIEN

"Where everything starts" will bring a proper 'END' to this book. It can't get crazier than that. I am inviting you back to the kitchen, as promised. To end something with the beginning is not crazier than starting with the end is ('Flashback' technique). This totally fits my crazy personality. So, let's *start to finish* the book. LOL

Here it is: Where everything starts is The Kitchen!

I heard this from many different healers so without a doubt**; where everything starts is in The Kitchen. Getting ill starts in the kitchen therefore getting healthy has to start in the kitchen, as well.**

You never thought that you only need good water for drinking, I hope?! It is also important to use good water for cooking. Cooking is a new, totally different experience when you have a Kangen® machine.

Thankfully, in British Columbia, more and more restaurants are also using Kangen Water®. More and more stores starting to sell organic, plant based wholesome foods.

Do you like food? I come from a family where everyone is a fan of good food but I think I am the one who is the most obsessed with it. I was born this way. My mom told me that she had to hide the bottle before she pushed it into my mouth as I got so crazily 'excited' just by spotting food that I could not swallow it properly. Yes, this is how I was as a baby and it did not change much in 65 years.

"We all eat, and it would be a sad waste of opportunity to eat badly."

ANNA THOMAS

To eat well is a requirement I think and not a luxury of some sort. We need good, quality food and the best nutrition to be healthy. I am not talking about different diet trends or indulging ourselves. Nothing like that. No one wants to eat bad food. No one wants a home full of chemicals. The majority, however, are struggling due to a poisonous lifestyle advertised for decades. I remember when I came to Canada ages ago, every second commercial on TV was advertising a different chemical. From air fresheners to candles, from bath tub cleaners to oven cleaners, everything was pushed with great success. Women loved it. My daughter and I, we just laughed, as we did not trust these chemicals or the commercials pushing them. This craziness had a real impact on our health and on our environment. Times are changing however. This nonsense has to stop.

Quite a few of us, who are inspired about a better way of life are trying hard to change the culture. People are talking a lot about being green or eco-friendly but really, what are the possibilities? How can we start to change things and start moving in the right direction? Probably many would appreciate the state-of-the-art 'helper' I have in my kitchen to experience 'the best' when it comes to food preparation, cooking, eating and living green. Some do have it but they have never been educated or have not taken the time to learn about the many different uses of the waters.

I have good news for all who care:

"You don't need a silver fork to eat good food."

PAUL PRUDHOMME

No, you don't. All you need is a Kangen® machine. What a difference we experienced when we started cooking with Kangen Water®. OMG!

Kids in general avoid veggies as they are alkaline and they can really taste the acidity of the poisons on the fruits and vegetables. These will not be washed off by tap water no matter how hard you try. I am saying this to help you with the difficult task of providing clean food for yourself and your family. Ever since I moved to this country, I have never been satisfied with the 'taste' of different foods. It just wasn't the same experience I had with food back home when I was growing up. And I am not alone! That changed with the waters from my Kangen® machine and it was a drastic change. Why or how, you might ask? Here it is: Most of the food we purchase has been sprayed, picked, packaged, shipped, sprayed again and stored for days, weeks or months before we bring it home.

There are things we need to consider before we consume the foods we eat, I learned. First, we have the people who have handled the produce (from pickers to cashiers). Secondly, as soon as a fruit or vegetable has been picked, it begins to decay and oxidize. Kangen Water® can effectively clean and revitalize your foods, reverse the effects of oxidation and significantly reduce spoilage. What do I mean when I talk about clean food? The same thing I mean when I talk about natural water. I don't want any additives, chemicals, poisons, pesticides, fungicides made from heavy metals or synthetic matter on my food. I don't want to waste food, either. You can save money and waste next to nothing. I like that. To waste food when so many are hungry is a terrible thing in itself.

Fruits and veggies can be disinfected, cleaned from pesticides, alkalised and revitalised with these waters. Meats can be soaked to eliminate harmful sodium and nitrates. Bacteria like salmonella, for

The Purple Wave

example, will be killed in less than five minutes with our 2.5 pH acidic water without killing us in the process. The 11.5 pH water is also a meat tenderiser. Sprayed chemicals can be completely removed from all produce. The difference in taste and experience is day and night. Everything cooks faster in Kangen Water®, in almost half the time and that will reduce the time of preparation and the energy used. Beans and grains, lentils, rice and nuts... etc. all need to be washed off from the sprayed chemicals. Most of this stuff is not washable by regular water, as they are oil based. From smoothies to salad dressings, we have special water for everything. Even your hardboiled eggs will be easier to peal the shell from if you know which water to use.

We are constantly hearing about food contamination and recalls. People are dying from foods. That is not normal. Food should be nourishing and enjoyable. We should create a food safety culture, not a food safety program.

Living a 'green' lifestyle has become a trendy topic in some circles, thank God. Ethically produced, packaged, recyclable foods should be taken into consideration.

What do you think about gardening? Gardening is the eco-friendliest activity. It is also great for health and the budget. It is good for the soul. It is connecting with nature, it is light exercise, it is what we all need. By gardening, we reduce needless waste, transportation costs, contamination, packaging materials, which are killing our trees and forests.

"We might think we are nurturing our garden, but of course it's our garden that is nurturing us."

JENNY UGLOW

Gardening is great by itself but it is even better and an absolute blessing when you have a Kangen® device. Plants can have remarkable 'hydration', nourishment and growth. The water from the machine will revitalize weak plants, help germination and it is chlorine free. This is also a great way to use the 'by-product waters' which come out from the secondary tube while you are producing drinking water for yourself.

I enjoy the flowers from my garden as those are the only ones, which are not loaded with pesticides nowadays. Most flowers, which you buy, don't even have a fragrance anymore so they don't work for me. Just as water should do its job to hydrate and detox the cells, flowers should fill up the air with amazing fragrances, not smelly stuff, which requires a gas mask. What has this world come to?

We are destroying the natural qualities of plants and fruits. We are trying to create fragrances with chemicals, after killing the natural fragrance. Of course, it doesn't work. As a consequence, these perfumes are banned at government offices, doctor's offices and they should be banned everywhere, period, as they are toxic. People have serious allergic reactions to them. It is not friendly to us. It is not organic. Our toxic cleaners made with chemicals smell like 'oranges' and our oranges smell like rat poison or pesticides. I hope you can see it now that we did indeed inherit an upside-down world.

When you have this technology, gardening goes to an all new level. For special plants, which prefer different pH waters, you can choose the most soothing pH from 4.5 to 11.5. There are plants which might need neutral water depending on the pH of the soil. Others love slightly alkaline, yet most prefer acidic waters. You can request your own guide in case you want to maximize you gardening abilities because as I said it before, we have it all.

> *"Food can destroy the world, but*
> *food can also heal it.*
> *The change starts with you."*
>
> **JOEL FUHRMAN M.D.**

Yes, Dr. Fuhrman. It is quite simple. We got it. Is this air-tight logic or what? I have no doubts about this statement. Do you?

The savings are also significant because of the endless possibilities to replace chemicals with just plain waters of different pH.

Some of the things which we replaced in our household are: makeup remover, window cleaner, hand sanitizer, rubbing alcohol, detergents, bug spray, pain killers, aspirin, vegetable wash, water softener, dishwasher detergent, cold or flu medications. The things we replaced in the kitchen and hardly ever buy them anymore are most of the minerals, digestive enzymes, soft drinks, bottled water, lemonade, fruit juices, homeopathic remedies, antibiotics, ointments, allergy medications... etc.

"Beware of little expenses, a small leak will sink a great ship."

BENJAMIN FRANKLIN

You will be able to save about forty percent on coffee and 80 percent on tea when you use the 9.5 water. Because of the different structure and penetrating ability of the water, the same strength of these beverages can be achieved with much less. There are tons of recipes already created but, of course, you can experiment and create some of your own. It is great fun. Oh, I should share my own. I created a lemonade recipe, which is refreshing, truly energising with no side effects (like coffee or energy drinks), and simple to make: 2 liters of Kangen®9.5 pH water, the juice of a whole organic lemon and ½ grapefruit (you can also use regular lemon or lime), 3-4 pieces of mint leaves, three table spoons of cane sugar. This lemonade is super detoxing and healthy. You can adjust the amount of lemon and sugar, to your taste.

With the help of our machine, eating 80 percent of your food raw (as we should) becomes 100 times easier and it won't appear to be such a crazy idea. I absolutely love veggies prepared the Kangen® way. It is exactly the way it was when I pulled out a carrot from my grandmother's organic garden 60 years ago or I ripped a totally organic fresh tomato off the vine. I still think that I am dreaming sometimes.

Cleaning also can be 'green'. We have to clean ourselves, our house, our laundry, our dishes, and on and on. "Indoor air pollution by hazardous chemicals is one of most serious environmental risks to human health", environmentalists are saying.

The majority of people don't like a dirty home but have a 'hazardous' home, instead.

So, what I am saying is, yes, it sounds crazy but a 'clean home' can be worse than a 'dirty home'. **I will call this a serious issue.** People are surprised why they are sick. According to recent study by *'Environmental Science and Technology in the USA'*, "*586 chemicals were identified in the American homes and 120 remained 'unidentified' by scientists*". Do you think this is important? So, get rid of the cleaners, detergents, beauty products, pet products, which are polluting your house and poisoning your family. This technology will do all that "naturally"! How is that possible? Well, a certified EPA testing lab recently tested the efficacy of the 2.5 pH Strong Acidic water made by the Enagic® Ioniser, as a sanitizer. The test demonstrated greater than 99.99 percent effectiveness to kill pathogens, like Salmonella, E-coli, Staph, MRSA, HIV, or the Hepatitis virus and much more. You won't find anything like this out there. This means that you are completely safe and you are better off staying home (not going to a hospital) with an infection like pink eye, a fungus, ingrown toe nail or anything of that sort. Wow. Yes, there is a way to live clean and green, once again. Please note that this water will only be potent for a maximum of two weeks, so yes you need a machine, you can't purchase this disinfectant water anywhere, because of the short shelf life!

"Don't call the world dirty because you forgot to clean your glasses!"

AARON HILL

Do you know places where you don't really want to go because you don't feel comfortable? I do. I avoid some people's houses because of smell, dog hair, lack of cleaning, toxic fragrances or the strong chemicals they use. I can't sleep in a bed where the bedsheets are washed with such a strong detergent that I can smell it all night long. Either, I won't fall asleep or I get a headache, which I never have otherwise.

"The objective of cleaning is not just to clean, but to feel happiness living within that environment."

MARIE KONDO

The Purple Wave

I know women who have beautiful kitchens but they hardly ever use them for cooking. How sad. To open cans, boxes and to eat frozen dinners, one doesn't need a $40,000 kitchen, only a can opener and a microwave. You don't need to buy it new, either, as garage sales are full of microwaves. Some smart people are trying to get rid of them.

I, myself, want to recognise my kids at age 95 if I live that long so I make my own food from fresh produce. I still clean my own house as I did all my life. My house and my kitchen are my business as a woman.

"My idea of superwoman is someone who scrubs her own floors!"

BETTE MIDLER

I used to be a 'superwoman' but I am not anymore. Dialysis, however, doesn't fit into my lifestyle so I choose to live a natural life. I don't have acrylic nails as I never did mind scrubbing the floors myself. Now Fred is doing all that stuff so I can finish this book. I know that we will experience some kind of 'ecstasy' for the first time when that happens.

The most common chemical compounds we successfully replaced in our household are mouthwash, make up remover, toner, air freshener, glass/window cleaners, laundry detergent, dishwasher soap (the 11.5 pH water won't leave any residue on the dishes). Stain removal has never been this easy and fun for me. Those kinds of chemicals have been all replaced in my laundry room just like the drying sheets with drying balls a long time ago. (Structure versus chemistry, right?) Less burden on our health and pocket. For the floors, we also have different waters, which work like a charm and even to clean a rug or the grout between the ceramic tiles is easy with the 11.5 pH water, which pulls dirt like nothing else. I love cleaning the bathroom with the three different waters I use. These are the 2.5, the 6.0 and the 11.5 pH waters.

We have recipes and instructions how to make detergent, air freshener, all those things. For air freshener, for example, I only use 'Beauty Water' from the machine and a few drops of essential oil. Cleaning the fridge has never been easier and absolutely no money spent on special, 'non toxic' cleaners.

The young moms are thrilled with the 2.5 pH water and how well it works for diaper rashes or any skin issues babies often have.

The Los Angeles Times recently ran an article about hotels (such as some of the Trump properties) in the US that are discovering the cost effectiveness of these waters and of course the housekeeping staff don't have to put up with the fumes of traditional cleaning chemicals.

They love it and they call it "El Miracle".

When it comes to skin care and personal care, in general, there is no debate that natural products are better to use but how much money are you willing to spend for the so-called 'organic' products? Most of them are very expensive. Thankfully, now you will have another alternative.

Eyebrows were raised when the huge Campaign for Safe Cosmetics in 2009 found that *"popular hair products including baby shampoo contained formaldehyde and other very toxic agents"*. Even the so called 'organic' products are only 70 percent natural as that is all that is required to be labelled as organic by federal requirements. Anyone want to know what is in the remaining thirty percent? I don't. I am done with the "organic dilemma'. I don't have to worry about it since I have my machine.

The different water protocols are extremely helpful for people with skin conditions. So many young people struggle with psoriasis, eczema, dermatitis or rashes - the label is not really important - because those are all signs of acidosis. I had psoriasis on my leg, which I could not get rid of for three years. I could not swim for three full winters as I had no skin on that part of my right leg from scratching. It can drive you crazy. I had a 'protocol' just to stop the itchiness every night, which lasted about half an hour; that meant scratching it until the skin came off completely and started bleeding. Then it started hurting more than the itchiness itself and that was easier to handle so I could actually fall asleep. Crazy memories, thankfully they are all in the past...

From rosacea to blisters and burns, from basic skin care to nasty and stubborn acne, from cuts, scrapes and wound care to herpes or serious diabetic gangrene, you can take care of these conditions by 'playing' with water.

Please watch the video on YouTube called, "Kangen Water® in Japanese Hospitals" to see how gangrene is solved 100 percent by the Kangen® machine. I personally know a gentleman who already was scheduled for amputation and the Kangen Water® protocol promoted by Hospitals in Japan and Korea reversed his condition. After one month, his doctor noticed the improvement and after another month his gangrene completely cleared, and his insulin requirement dropped to 50 percent. The stories are endless. We would like you to take this tool seriously. It is a much-needed device.

What do you think about antiperspirants? This is another billion-dollar industry!

*"One rumor in particular that antiperspirant use causes cancer received such interest that a number of cancer research and information organizations **were forced to post statements denying the link between breast cancer and the use of antiperspirants,**"* says Dr. Michael Greger, MD, on a video. Today we know that this is indeed true and that the many different uses of aluminum are quite hazardous to our health. Dr. Greger is the author of an amazing book called: "How Not to Die". The earliest suspicion of aluminium being very toxic was recorded when a story called "The mortician's mystery" surfaced. This was the inspiration for a group of researchers to see what is the truth about these toxic metallic agents. So, this has been known since the early 80s.

I hope that you got rid of your antiperspirant by now.

Toxic or not, sweating is important when it comes to getting rid of toxins. When you prevent that natural function, you are disabling your lymphatic system. Its main purpose is to keep the body from accumulation of toxins. Toxicity will bring acidosis and acidosis could lead to cancer. It is a very straightforward and logical process.

There are books and written material, which will show you the different protocols for how to live perfectly well without antiperspirants. One step at a time will bring you to a more natural lifestyle and you will restore your health. This is all part of that detox you need so badly. It won't happen in a week. In this process, the Kangen machine® will be your main tool.

The protocol for nasal lavage, for example, will help you if you have inflammation, mucosal lining problems, allergies, sinuses, snoring or sleep apnea.

Another common thing is periodontal disease or as some might call it, gingivitis. I have never seen a better remedy to stop that than our 2.5 pH water. I use it almost every day. To use this water is easy and effective. Acid reflux, constipation, food poisoning, it doesn't matter, can be resolved at home with very little effort.

There are easy to follow protocols for irritable bowel syndrome, which will probably disappear as soon as you start drinking the water, for yeast infections and more. I would whole heartedly recommend the book called "Ionized Water Protocols" by Dr. Peggy Parker. It is an amazing work.

Many owners don't maximize the use of this high-end unit. The 2.5 acidic water is a safe and natural alternative to stop HIV, Hepatitis, MRSA, E-coli, salmonella and other nasty bacteria and viruses, infections and helps with skin conditions like eczema, and psoriasis. Who wants to be without these waters? That would be reckless and irresponsible, especially these days.

"Your Home, a Chemical Free Sanctuary" by Peggy Parker is a great guide, which will teach you how to clean the house with water only. To be kind to the environment can be fun and very rewarding at the same time.

*"Only he who can see the invisible
can do the impossible."*

FRANK L. GAINES

AFTERTHOUGHTS

EVERYTHING YOU NEED

*"If you have a garden and a library, you
have everything you need."*

CICERO

L et me add Kangen Water® to that. So, we need three things. We
have so much more these days than a garden and a library and
most of these just complicate our lives. So we have everything but the
things which we really need. A strange and upside down situation, as we
mentioned it before. So, what can we do?

Dear friends. Never stop asking questions!

See the possibilities, see the invisible. Almost everything the water does
is invisible but we can give it a try, we can drink it, we can learn about it
and experience it. This way we see the invisible work of water and that
leads to impossible results. Some would never believe everything that
happened with us or what was possible in these seven years. Once you
have the 'foundation' for your health, good water, you can build on it with
confidence. You also got the 'secret ingredient' for the best tasting food.

Water remains a 'mystery' to most of us, of course, but almost
nothing is impossible if you are faithfully drinking Kangen Water®. Dr.

Barry Awe is another believer who has an amazing demo on YouTube. I had to see it five times. Barry is a chiropractor, whose health wasn't that great ever since he was a child and his young wife had cancer. Find it and see what is indeed possible with this water.

Creating this technology was obviously an international affair. Instead of fighting each other, people actually worked together.

I am sure that even Leonardo Da Vinci himself and Marie Curie, Einstein or Jacques Cousteau would approve this effort.

> **"Water and air, the two essential**
> **fluids on which life depends, have**
> **become global garbage cans."**
>
> **COUSTEAU**

Harsh words but they are needed to wake up this sleeping world. Jacques Cousteau (1910-1997) was born in France. He was an extraordinary explorer of nature. People beat themselves up because they had a drinking night or they enjoyed a chocolate bar. I usually just double my water intake and take some extra vitamin C if I had sweets I shouldn't have had. The antioxidant power of the water will take care of the oxidation and the acidity. It will take care of the extra stress. It will hydrate and help in restoring the immune system. It will make detoxing constant and easy and that leads to balance. This is the peace of mind I am talking about.

When Kangen Water® came into my life, I was so busy working, worrying about my health, pain, mortgages, bills, taxes, that in the never-ending process of 'making money' I almost lost sight of what was really important. I forgot that we always have to be open to possibilities as we never know when the biggest blessing is knocking on our door. I was kind of lonely up on the hill in my big house and overwhelmed with work. Soon after my health broke down, my finances followed.

The Purple Wave

"When you stop chasing the wrong things you give the right things a chance to catch you."

LOLLY DASKAL

The sooner you wake up to this fact, the better off you are.

There is a big difference between what we want and what we really need!

All I needed was water my body would accept and love. I almost missed it. I was very close to not trying the water or never going to a "water-presentation".

It isn't only me who missed what should be the centre of our focus. The scientific world missed it as well by "chasing the wrong things", following the wrong path. The worldwide system grabbed the 'germ theory' of Pasteur (1822-1895) because it fit their agenda. It gave Big Pharma a free pass to sell their drugs. Pasteur himself recognised that his theory was a 'mistake' before he died. That did not stop the medical establishment from adopting the theory as the truth, the whole truth and nothing but the truth. Dr. Gary Tunsky, ND, who is one of the world's leading experts on the subject of pH, states:

"Pasteur's 'Germ Theory' is a Hoax!"

"The adoption by science of Louis Pasteur's germ theory as the whole truth (that germs and pathogens are the direct cause of most disease), without regard to the deep insight of Antoine Bechamp's principle (that the acidic condition of the patient's cellular environment creates disease), marks one of the most dramatic and dynamic turns of events in modern history." Pasteur was a chemist, a biologist and a microbiologist, born in France. Antoine Bechamp (1816-1908) was another French scientist, a rival of Pasteur who had many breakthroughs in organic chemistry.

So, modern orthodox medicine arose upon a scientific error, which is this 'kill everything' mindset. Kill the bacteria, kill the virus, kill the fungus, and kill the tumor, which has played a major role in the promotion of illness by the creation of resistant strains of bacteria and the suppression of symptoms, not the reversal of illness.

It's not the bacteria or the viruses themselves that produce the disease. It's the chemical by-products of these microorganisms (free radicals and such) and the chemicals we bring into our system, acting upon the unbalanced, malfunctioning cell metabolism of the human body that in actuality creating disease. If the body's cellular metabolism and pH is perfectly balanced, it is susceptible to no illness or disease. Once again, we should provide the right terrain or environment in our cells.

This eleven-year-old girl, crippled with arthritis did not need meds, pills, antibiotics or anything of that sort. She was probably extremely acidic, by drinking sodas. She only needed structured water to get out of the wheelchair. She was blessed by meeting Dr. Don Colbert who offered her this water. I heard this story by listening to a CD, called: "The amazing Health machine." Dr. Colbert is a famous doctor who is getting lots of media coverage these days. He is recognised and very much loved by the Christian Community in the United States and Canada. Almost everyone I talk to knows him or his books. Elvis Stojko did not need anything but this water to avoid or prevent knee replacements, hip replacements and all the rest. By his own testimony, most of his Olympic colleges are having these issues. Not him. At age 45 he is still capable of doing what he did all his life. He has been drinking Kangen Water® for over ten years now. Wow.

When someone starts and keeps drinking this water faithfully, their body will talk to them and that is the ultimate experience you need so no one can 'talk you out' of drinking water.

> ### *"Man's mind, once stretched by a new idea, never regains its original dimensions."*
>
> **OLIVER W. HOLMES**

Through a European connection of mine I recently came into contact with a very special physiotherapist. This man is Ming Chew from New York. He is not your usual therapist. He, himself, was a body builder and an athlete. He developed the "Ming' method for healing after injury. There is a good reason why he is more successful with world class athletes than doctors or surgeons. Chew understands the 'Fascia-Pain' connection. He also gets the injury and dehydration connection. His book is remarkable.

The Purple Wave

He is actually teaching people how to do the therapy themselves so they don't have to rely on him or other therapists. This is a real healer. A healer has to be a teacher, as well. People need help. I think this is marvellous as nowadays we have millions who are seeking help after car accidents, sport and other injuries. They need rehabilitation, which actually works.

One of Chew's patients was NBA star, Jason Kidd. He actually put him back to the sport after conventional doctors could not do anything for him. This expert knows that when it comes to pain, dehydration is the big issue. He states: *"Most Medical professionals believe that injuries, aches and pains can be fixed by medication or surgery. I do this by treating a little-known tissue called the fascia."* The fascia envelopes every muscle, tendon, nerve and organ in the body. This sensitive protective membrane is filled with nerve endings. Of course, it hurts when dried out or dehydrated. Apparently masters of shiatsu acupuncture or chiropractors and other practitioners don't necessarily pay attention to the tightness of the fascia. Chew says that *"the fascia has to be actively stretched. Before that happens, it has to be very well hydrated"*. Chew and many others don't know about our super hydrating water. I asked him and he uses other kinds. Not for long. He aims to help his patients to recover 100 percent. He mentioned in his book that indeed it bothers him that he himself has not been able to recover 100 percent from his own injury. When we use this tool with compassion, we are changing the world. I have no doubt about that. That is our part. Why not to do it? Compassion is a beautiful and extremely rewarding exercise.

> **"I think technology really increased human ability.**
> **But technology cannot produce compassion."**
>
> **DALAI LAMA**

I know that our water will give everyone maximum results. Let me tell you the story of another friend. She suffered a car accident fifteen months before we met. Tons of multiple therapy paid by the insurer for all this period could not help her in getting rid of pain. She was told that there is nothing they can do for her. She was having mostly sleepless nights for over a year and naturally could not function the next day. In one month, soon after she started drinking Kangen Water®, she was feeling much better; her pain just went away and indeed never came back. She told me the amazing news. Ira is a successful distributor now, just another person who got her life back. I got much more back from Ira than I gave to her. This is how this plays out most of the time.

What a tool we have on our hands! What a tool and what a blessing! Thank you, Mr. 'O', and thank you all who have put effort into this marvellous idea.

I believe that the very reason why people get injured at times is that this very thin membrane dries out. Oh no, do we have a new discovery again? I don't mind as long as we can finish this book!

Apparently (an expert opinion, not mine), migraines are also the consequence of a dried out fascia, or 'membrane'. What happens with migraines is that the 'meninges' (membrane which covers the brain) becomes dehydrated and starts tightening almost to the point of breaking causing that tremendous pain. The brain has no nerve, or nerve endings, so it is obvious that the brain itself can't become 'painful'. I believe this theory. It makes sense but here's the proof: We had a woman who missed more days from work than days she could work because of the tremendous migraine pains she used to have. She reacted so well to the water that her migraines completely ceased in a month and never returned. I never had migraines myself, which is a miracle in itself but I feel bad to see this issue so many are having. People take pain killers for migraine headaches. If hydration won't take care of this problem, you might need a good chiropractor to see if you need some kind of adjustment.

What a brilliant example of what we spoke about before. We are treating the symptoms in today's dumbed down society and we don't address the cause. Avicenna would end up in the mental institution if he was alive today just like Dr. Semmelweis did.

With this last testimony, the stories end but only in this book. Life goes on and a wonderful new chapter waits for all who embrace this lifestyle.

I have tried my best to share everything I learned, experienced or witnessed. I did this with love and integrity, with respect towards our Creator, our environment, this beautiful Earth and the human race, which includes You.

My "prescription" (which should never get me in trouble) for you is this: Despite the weather forecast, live like the Sun always is shining on you but also love the rain. I do. The rain is beautiful, it is water for the earth. We all need it.

> *"The best thing one can do when*
> *it is raining is to let it rain."*
>
> **HENRY W. LONGFELLOW**

The amount of water we recommend (it brings unbelievable results when you faithfully do it) is one-half an ounce per pound per day per body weight. Do this for two or three weeks and watch what happens! For example, if you weigh 160 pounds, you should drink four liters of Kangen Water® every twenty-four hours. If you are doing rigorous exercise or heavy-duty physical activity, you will require more. If you are drinking lots of coffee you will need even more.

Further, I am not prescribing only suggesting that you love yourself first by taking care of your body and spirit.

Learn from the stories/testimonials and from the many lessons of history. Read some books. There is tremendous wealth in books; wealth, which is much more valuable than money. Good books and Nature are places where you can go and collect 'nectar', just like the bees.

'Ride The Purple Wave', drink Kangen® 9.5, the only water people should be drinking" as Shan Stratton, this top nutritionist claims this at every one of his demos filled with passion.

Transform your home into a "chemical free sanctuary". It is up to you how far you want to go with this new, green life. It is your life and your family's life. Care much more about yourself and much less about what others might think or say.

When you are spiritually and physically strong, love, peace, happiness, fulfillment or joy will become real and reachable to you!

What else do you need?

Spread the word about water! Be smart, be your own doctor, a scientist, an artist whoever you want to be, but before anything else: Be yourself!

Trust the amazing substance that natural water is and trust your own, truly amazing immune system. Be confident, after all, you just found a new art for prevention, vitality, performance and longevity.

Oh, I should caution you: If you are drinking Kangen Water®, make sure your adult children are drinking it, as well, otherwise a strange situation might occur. You might look better and younger than them and who would want that to happen?

At times, I come across people who are 'very smart' like extremely smart, you know. They say; "if the water is so great and is medical grade, we should only drink it when we get sick." This makes me laugh so hard as I used to laugh only during my teenage years. (You remember that crazy laugh, don't you?) I don't see or find any logic in that nonsense. I tell you why. It is easier, much easier to prevent an illness than to get rid of it. Medical grade water does not bear the same idea as a medically prescribed drug. Indeed. It refers to its tremendous therapeutic value and preventative nature. Period. For all of you, 'nuclear scientists', keep it simple!

This crazy mindset created by an ill society is too painful even to think about.

How do you see Kangen Water® now? Are you celebrating?

This is how I see it:

"Every good and perfect gift
comes from above."

James 1.17

The Purple Wave is the wave of the Future!

Hopefully, we will not poison the life of the seas and the rest of this beautiful Earth much longer. The future begins when our morals and responsibilities, not money or profits, start guiding us.

The benefits of a Kangen® machine are endless. No book is big enough to list all its possible uses. The applications of the different grades of water are now in hospitals all over the Orient. It has been present in hospitals all over Japan for forty years now. The best known hospitals are: Kyowa Hospital, Kitari Institute Medical Center, Showa University Hospital,

The Purple Wave

Meiseki Hospital, Hanabatake Hospital, the Tokyo Women's College of Medicine and many others. Japan has been the number one country for health, longevity and common sense for a long time. Hopefully, a change in lifestyle and some progress towards a better future will happen soon here on the American continents and all over Europe, as well. We have numerous veterinary doctors, physicians, chiropractors, Natural Health Practitioners and dentists who are using Kangen® machines already, with great success and results.

"God and Nature first made us what we are,
and then out of our own created genius we make
ourselves what we want to be. Follow
always that great law..."

MARCUS GARVEY

Diets, fasting, colonics and many different detox techniques people used during history all have become popular for a good reason. If you have any doubts at all regarding the fantastic benefits of detoxing or illnesses being the consequences of getting 'filthy' inside, this should help you. I am sure you heard about 'epilepsy' and how horrible this "illness" is. There are over 300,000 kids at the moment living in the USA alone who are suffering and probably drugged under the label called 'epilepsy'. I think that these kids (most of them anyway), these beautiful human beings suffer in vain because they are dehydrated and have a dirty and toxic body and brain.

What you might not know is that a special diet called the "Ketogenic diet" developed by Russel Wilder in 1921 at the Mayo clinic in the United States is working wonderfully for 'epileptic children'. The results are so amazing that this 'diet'- combined with fasting, which brings some metabolic changes to the body - is used now by 75 centres, in forty-five countries. This info is, of course, supressed (no one can say that these kids are cured); still just by 'word of mouth' (just like Kangen Water®) many are discovering this well-hidden natural therapy.

My question is this: How come detoxing with this diet works so well for all these people? Again, if something turned out to be such a great solution, it must be addressing the exact cause! What this tells me is this: Hundreds of thousands of kids are not really sick, but 'dirty' at the cellular level, their brain is in 'crisis' situation just like that man's brain was we saw at the restaurant. In case you think I am crazy - again - there is a TV drama made in 1997, directed by Jim Abrahams, called, "First Do No Harm!" The movie is really a documentary about the accurate and true story of a sweet little boy, one of the many people who used this special diet for three years and completely recovered from the horrible condition often labelled as "epilepsy". Suffering from 'severe epilepsy', the kid was completely unresponsive to medications. These pills had terrible side effects and the family was exhausted from taking care of him. There was no hope for them when the mother in her despair and agony finds the information about this diet, in a book, at the library. She goes through the 'fight of her life' to get the child out of the hospital and get him accepted by this clinic. Her son recovered 100 percent by following the diet and all meds are dropped, of course. Wow. How crazy all things in this system have gotten. How can we ignore information this vital? I think we found the answer. The 'craziness' we have to deal with on a daily basis is not unintentional. There are many who live quite well by keeping millions (the majority) in the dark.

*"**A few thousands of 'epileptics', who cleaned themselves out, by the so called "Ketogenic diet ", now live totally symptom free, without seizures***" is told at the end of the documentary. How this film was possible without funding or advertising is interesting. I find it heart-warming. Most of the 'actors' are real people "not cured" but made completely well from "disease" by this diet. Am I politically correct enough? Not that I care...

How much easier it is to keep yourself clean by using Kangen Water®, plenty of water, I am thinking.

Will it make sense to you to drink water, which is cleansing at the cellular level? If you only prevent something labelled as epilepsy, it is worth having this water in your house. Case closed!

How easy it is to miss the most important things in life when we are not really listening!

It all depends on us! It all depends on you. If you want to be healthy, do something about it!

Your life will get better by choice and not by chance.

Now you've got another tool. I should say; now you've got the *main* tool to make your life better and easier.

The Purple Wave

At this time in history we don't need smarter people, we need healthy people. Therefore, I don't recommend to you to become a scientist by searching and researching. I recommend you drink the water and become healthy, healthier than ever before.

> ***"I believe that the greatest gift you can give your family and the world is a healthy YOU."***
>
> **JOYCE MEYER**

Every single person who I know, who has been successful with their own healing, understood that their courage, patience and determination was the big idea that turned them around towards a better life. This determination of course included other lifestyle changes as well, not only drinking quality water.

As Sam, a scientist friend of mine, who calls himself a 'recovering scientist' likes to say, *"research is only re-search"*. When he found Kangen Water®, he found what he was "searching for" so he stopped searching and researching all together.

I find this absolutely marvellous.

"Enhancing the quality and properties of the water consumed will improve hydration at the cellular level, thus helping the body maintain balance, facilitate healing and regeneration. Consumption of acidic and denatured foods brings the production of mucus, which over time develops into a 'mucoid' plague. This is the body's response and coping mechanism to protect itself. It is critical to have regular cleansing so the elimination pathways of the body are cleared for optimal functioning. " Very eloquently expressed by Byron Scheffler an exceptional professional from Vancouver, BC, I met during my research. Byron is a Live Blood Analysis expert with great integrity and the president of Inherent Wellness. He understands and reassures us that "the symptoms can be alleviated by shifting one's paradigm, focusing on the fundamentals." These are a clean, balanced, functioning mind and body. This is how we avoid health complications, the exact opposite of what conventional, main stream medicine does. These unwanted complications are limitless and will end with unbearable dis-eases. Byron himself is another witness to these simple and natural approaches, as he casted aside the main stream approaches when he experienced health challenges, just like I did.

You can still go and research but please avoid Google as that 'exercise' will only make your head spin. To properly research ERW, again, please go to www.PubMed.gov

The only thing (there is always one exception, right?) which did not improve with the water is my funny 'European accent'. Or maybe it did? If you did not notice it, the water did 'cure' it. I should not use this word 'cure' as this word seems forbidden. No one is allowed to use it! I am denying that my accent is gone, okay? It is true. As soon as you call me, you will hear it.

I love Enagic® as a company. I love everything the machine does.

I know that you will love it, too. How do I know? It is quite simple; there is nothing not to like about it.

"Enagic" is a new 'word'. Everyone is asking me, what is it? This is the story; Enagic is a combination of two words: energy and magic.

Energy + Magic = Enagic. Got it? I heard this from the' lion's mouth'. Mr. 'O' came up with it, himself.

Mr. Ohshiro is not only an exceptionally good man with a brilliant mind, but he is also an exceptional diplomat. He never says that our water helps with depression or anything else. He calls it, 'happy water'. There is much more truth and wisdom in these two words than people might think.

**"The most important thing in communication
is hearing what isn't said."**

PETER DRUCKER

This is true in life in general but even more so when it comes to Kangen Water®! If you grew up in a society like I did, a communist dictatorship where there is zero freedom of speech, you learn how to read between the lines. You do that to survive. I learned that total freedom of speech is not necessarily given in other forms of society, either. It must have been limited in ancient times, as well, because the

The Purple Wave

truth was hidden in proverbs and different writings. **Truth is likely to arise from 'hidden' sources.** I 'heard' and easily understood everything that wasn't said about Kangen Water®. So, the best is if we don't talk too much. We just give out the water with love and we drink it with faith. Get near to a source as soon as possible so you can experience it yourself. It took me years to play with it and to grasp how significant this whole idea and technology is. Often, I can't take my mind off this amazing water. The very purpose of this book is to share it and show it to as many people as I can. The good but rare 'habit' of drinking water is insanely important.

What we need is a positive mindset and a negative charge. This is another secret formula to a healthy life!

It is up to you now what you think or believe about Kangen Water®. What you've got here is ancient science and modern technology.

I called this a 'marriage made in heaven'.

This is my story, a short version of it. This is how I became really rich, extremely rich. I became richer in my thinking, in my physical body and in my soul. I am royalty now. It is okay if you don't agree. Not everyone will agree, because...

> *"Health is the crown on the*
> *well person's head that only*
> *the ill person can see."*
>
> **ROBIN SHARMA**

The most significant secret to health is that the solution, the answer resides within you. You just have to take responsibility.

Please let me know if this long story of the many short stories made it easier for you to recognise the unique value of this technological marvel and the significance of this therapeutic water. I consider great ideas and fabulous discoveries, which serve all of us, (rather than only special interest groups) a blessing. We need to implement ideas in our lives, which are proven by time, not by data only, I believe.

I am forever grateful for Kangen Water® and I will make sure that every drop counts.

Thank you for staying with me to the end. Please do not hesitate to contact me for help or more information.

In case there is someone who cared enough to share the water, some information or this book with you, please contact them to get your unit hooked up in your home, as soon as possible. That is the Enagic® way, and the ethical way.

We, the sometimes overly passionate Kangen family, the guards of this water, wish you and your family great physical health, even greater mental health and peace of mind, which comes with financial health.

I am available on FB, as Klara Reid. You can also email me at: ecolifeandpassionredefined@gmail.com or check out our web-page: LifeAndPassionRedefined.com

Simple definitely wins in this complicated world!

Simplicity, however, is not a new idea. It has been and will always be part of a great life, eternal wisdom and joy.

There is nothing on Earth as amazing as the Grace of God. I understand this now with absolutely no difficulty. The grace that was poured on me is much more than I deserve....

"Grace is finding a waterfall when you were only looking for a stream."

VANESSA HUNT

Yes, the 'girl' needed water and she was blessed by the best water there is.

This is how my personal story of chronic dehydration and the amazing story of Kangen Water® came together. I hope you have been inspired through these revelations and work. Let's share this with many more wonderful people on this beautiful Earth.

And now, the mountains are calling, the rivers are rolling, the birds are singing, and the Sun is shining, I've got to go...

Klara, with a *"K"*

"THERE IS NO GREATNESS WHERE
THERE IS
NO SIMPLICITY, GOODNESS
AND TRUTH."

LEO TOLSTOY

REFERENCE LIBRARY

DR. HIROMI SHINYA M.D. -The Enzyme Factor
DR. HIROMI SHINYA M.D. -The Rejuvenation Enzyme
DR. BATMANGHELIDJ M.D. -You're Not Sick, You're Thirsty
DR. BATMANGHELIDJ M.D. -Your Body's Many Cries for Water
DR. MICHAEL R. LYON M.D. -Is Your Child's Brain Starving?
DR. TIM MCNIGHT M.D. N.D.-Confessions of a Skeptical Physician
DR. DAVE CARPENTER. N.D. -Change Your Water ... Change Your Life
RON GARNER N.D. -After the Doctors...What Can You Do?
SUSANNAH CAHALAN - Brain on Fire
ROBERT G. WRIGHT -Killing Cancer Not People
DR. JERRY TENNANT M.D.-Healing is Voltage
WADE T LIGHTHEART, KATRINE VOLYNSKY-Staying Alive in a Toxic World
DR. H.S. FILTZER, M.D.- Kangen Water®, Scientific Study Results on the Benefits of Kangen Water®
DR.MU SHIK JHON-The Water Puzzle and the Hexagonal Key
DR. W. GIFFORD-JONES M.D. 90+, How I Got There
DR. BERNARD JENSEN D.C.PH.D.- Tissue Cleansing through Bowel Management
DR. T. BAROODY M.D. -Alkalize or Die
SHERRY A. ROGERS -Detoxify or die
DAN BUETTNER. -Blue Zones-Lessons for Living Longer from the People Who've Lived the Longest
Dr. RALPH CINQUE -Quit for good: How to break a bad habit
Suzie Derrett -All shook up, my natural fight against cancer
TOSHIO MAEHARA -Success Story
HIRONARI OHSHIRO Quenching the Thirst for Global Success
DR. LENKEI GABOR M.D. – Censored health.
DR. LENKEI GABOR M.D.- A betegseg ipar futoszallagan, A koleszterin

nem artalmas

GERALD L. KOSTECKA - Ride the Wave

DR. LADD R. MCNAMARA M.D. -The Cholesterol Conspiracy

DR. MYRON WENTZ PH. D. - Invisible Miracles

MING CHEW – The Permanent Pain Cure

DR. MICHAEL GREGER M.D -How Not to Die.

DR. CORINNE ALLEN N.D. -The Science and Practical Uses of ERW in Brain and Neurological Issues [DVD]

VALERIE GREENE -Conquering Stroke: How I fought my way back and how you can too.

DR. PEGGY PARKER- Ionised Water Protocols, Your Home... A Chemical Free Sanctuary, Using Ionised Water in the Kitchen

Dr. T. Colin Campbell -The China study

YouTube Documentaries:

Roger Gaudette presentations and Demos

World of Hydration

- Water, the great mystery.
- Water, natural salt and exercise in that order, Dr. Batmangehidj
- Escape Fire: The fight to Rescue American Healthcare.
- The disappearing male
- Dr. Barry Awe. Kangen demo
- Dr. Michael talks about Kangen water (2015 Revised)
- Kangen Water® in Japanese Hospitals
- Sharyl Attkisson -Astroturf and Manipulation on Media Messages
- First do no harm! - Producer Jim Abrahams
- Dr. Michael talks about Kangen Water® (2015 revised)
- GPM-Kangen Water® Demo with Bob Gridelli and Elvis Stojko
- 2-time Olympic Silver medalist and World Figure Skating Champion Elvis Stojko on Kangen Water®

Netflix documentary: Game changers

ALL BIBLE QUOTES ARE FROM THE NEW WORLD TRANSLATION of the HOLY SCRIPTURES.